THE
GOD-AWAKENING
DIET

Reversing disease
and saving the planet
with a
plant based diet

AQIYL ANIYS

ISBN-13: 978-1530991846
ISBN-10: 1530991846
CreateSpace Independent Publishing Platform, North Charleston, SC

ACKNOWLEDGEMENT

Thanks to "The Unity" and "Sustainer of Life" for letting me grow to understand the tremendous awesomeness of your oneness a little bit more.

CONTENTS

THE GOD-AWAKENING DIET

CHAPTER 1:

CONNECTIVITY

I have encountered much more than I had ever expected while on my plant-based-diet journey. My journey had become so eye-opening that it led me to become a plant-based-diet health activist. My journey started as an attempt to improve my health and led to an expected increase in energy, endurance, mental clarity, and emotional well-being, as well as a greater connection to the world around me. My plant-based journey has helped to remove the *I* from me and has strengthened my conscious connection to that which unifies life.

This unification is conceptualized in various ways, and to reduce the likeliness of argument, I will refer to this unifying force as God/The Source/Nature. My simple change in diet is responsible for me viewing the world and life as a unified force made up of many parts that naturally work together with synergy. This connectivity and synergy is represented in natural patterns that some recognize and few truly understand.

An example of this is the way birds fly in a *V* pattern. It is undeniably very beautiful that a flock of birds can synchronize and fly in this pattern, and they are able to do this without the level of intelligence that humans have. Scientific studies have discovered that these birds interact and flow with air currents generated by the flapping of their wings.[1] As the bird in front flaps its wings, it generates upward currents of airflow behind it. The bird that is behind that bird will fly in

1

that current, which gives that bird a lift; it doesn't have to work as hard to fly. This allows the bird that is behind to conserve energy. The bird that is in front will switch positions with the bird or birds that are behind, and this will allow the bird in front to also rest and conserve energy.

The birds reveal the natural patterns that are generated by the flapping of their wings, and they work with and use the patterns to generate more efficient work than they would if they were flying by themselves. The birds are able to fly longer distances than if they were flying solo because they are able to conserve more energy by flying in the upward currents. There is no separation between the birds and the air they fly through, and when they work with the forces of God/The Source/Nature as a unit, they produce synergy in their work; they accomplish more than they would on their own.

These subtle patterns of connectivity and interdependence exist throughout all of life, but we often overlook them. Our relationship to the sun comes to mind when I think about how we overlook this connectivity. The sun plays an extremely important role in supporting our vitality and homeostasis, but today, in most of our societies, the sun is just an object in the sky that gives light to the day. In the ecosystem of the world we live in, the sun is much more than that. It is known that the sun is vital to the life of plants. Plants convert sunlight into chemical energy through a process called photosynthesis, to supply plants with food.[2]

Many people don't realize the sun is as important for human health as it is for the health of plants. Our natural source of vitamin D is attained through our special relationship to the sun. Our bodies produce vitamin D naturally when our bodies absorb UVB radiation from sunlight. This produces a chemical reaction in the skin that transforms cholesterol in the body into vitamin D. Our natural connectivity to the sun is vitally important for us maintaining homeostasis in the body.[3, 4] Homeostasis is the tendency toward a relatively stable equilibrium between interdependent elements, and the body continuously works toward accomplishing that state.

Homeostasis is equated with health, and the body works to maintain this state of health by using natural elements and compounds derived from the ecosystem we are a part of to fuel and maintain cell health. Vitamin D is one these compounds and may very well be the most important compound for sustaining homeostasis in the body.[5]

This vitamin that is provided to us easily and freely by just being in the grace of God/The Source/Nature's sunlight, does so much more for our overall health than science previously supported. Traditional medicine has been aware of the special relationship of humans to the sun and its support of our mental and physical health. African cultures, like the ancient Egyptian dynasties and their depictions of sun gazers, attest to this understanding.

Until recently, Western science focused mostly on vitamin D's role in helping the body absorb calcium in supporting bone health and strength. Scientific studies now show that vitamin D is involved in much more than this, which has led to revised recommendations.

New scientific studies show that vitamin D deficiency has been linked to an increased risk of death from cardiovascular disease, asthma, cognitive impairment like Alzheimer's disease, autoimmune disease like multiple sclerosis, cancer, chronic inflammatory diseases, Crohn's disease, depression, hypertension, and type 1 and type 2 diabetes. God/The Source/Nature has provided us with the healing power of sun to help us avoid these diseases, but we have lost sight of this connectivity and now actually run away from the sun. We run away from the sun with good reason. The industries we develop destroy the natural balance of our earth's ecosystem that God/The Source/Nature has given to all life on earth.

Our atmosphere was balanced with elements and compounds that allowed in just the right amount of radiation and heat to support the ecosystem that developed on the planet earth. Human intervention has disrupted that balance by developing products and industries that release pollution containing chlorofluorocarbons (CFCs) and hydrochlorofluorocarbons (HCFCs) into the atmosphere that deplete the protective ozone layer.[6, 7] Giving way to technology and industrial advances over understanding and protecting the natural patterns that exist in life has its repercussions. The depletion of the ozone layer results in increased risk of skin cancer and malignant-melanoma development humans and animals. The depletion also results in tree, plant, and marine-life damage.[8]

We live in or are influenced by a technical and industrial Western-dominant paradigm that is focused on manipulating natural patterns of life, often at the expense of the natural God/The Source/Nature patterns that already exist. The paradigm's influence is so strong that we often overlook or pay little attention to the natural patterns that exist right in front of our faces, patterns that we are a part of.

My adoption of a plant-based diet is greatly responsible for my change in paradigm from seeing myself as apart from God/The Source/Nature to seeing myself as a part of God/The Source/Nature. Seeing myself as part of the connectivity and synergy of life involved a leap of faith spearheaded by the philosophy of the herbalist Dr. Sebi. It was a leap of faith because the knowledge of traditional medicine founded on the healing power of plants was also hidden for me by a reductionist paradigm geared toward promoting research that isolates properties of components with the purpose of developing technology, ultimately for economic gain. This paradigm supports research that will produce technology for economic gain over research that will prove the natural healing ability of plants, which would ultimately cut into the profits made from selling technology. The truth often becomes muddied in this process, which often makes it difficult to find the real truth when it comes to nutrition and healing.

The consumption and promotion of meat protein is a prime example. The alarming increase in meat consumption is greatly responsible for the destruction of our ecosystem as well as the destruction of our bodies, which I like to refer to as the temple of God/The Source/Nature. As a global society, our increased meat production and consumption is directly and indirectly the most destructive thing to the natural God/The Source/Nature patterns established in our bodies and in the world.

I know this might seem farfetched, but let's take a look at the development of the meat industry, our constructed paradigms about the importance of animal protein, and the way the politics, economics, and manipulation of scientific research destroys our health and the world around us.

CHAPTER 2:

EXCESS ANIMAL PROTEIN DESTROYS THE BODY

I started this vegan journey by accepting the methodology and philosophy of herbalist Dr. Sebi that plant-based foods were healing foods and animal-based foods were not. Non-GMO and non-hybrid-plant-based foods alkalized and produced an environment in the body that was inhospitable to disease. Animal-based foods and unwhole plant foods acidified the body and provided a hospitable environment for disease to thrive. I ended up diving into his methodology, adopted a plant-based diet, and was on my way toward healing myself and rejuvenating my body.

While I was well along my plant-based journey, I participated in Dr. Colin Campbell's plant-based-nutrition certificate program, and it corroborated the herbalist Dr. Sebi's view about the detrimental effect that the overconsumption of animal protein has on the body. Dr. Colin Campbell was previously an avid promoter of the consumption of animal-based protein as a way of combating malnutrition in the world most economically. He also developed the great epidemiological study, the China Project, which opened his eyes to the benefits of a whole-food, plant-based diet. Dr. Colin Campbell's studies on animal-based and plant-based protein and the China Project made it clear to him that animal-based protein was not the savior he thought it to be.

The course pointed out that the heavy promotion of the consumption of animal-based protein was ignited by a study done in 1914.[9] The researchers studied the effects of rats' consumption of animal-based proteins and plant-based proteins. They noticed the rats grew more rapidly while eating animal-based proteins, and other studies during the time resulted in the same conclusions. It was concluded that animal-based proteins were superior to plant-based proteins, because plant-based proteins were thought to lack sufficient amounts of certain amino acids to properly support normal growth. This placed the focus on animal-based protein as being the most important nutrient in supporting health.

Though plants contained the amino acids we needed, they did not contain them in the ratio that supported quick synthesis and fast growth. Since animal-based proteins have a similar makeup to our own proteins, the body synthesizes them more easily promoting faster growth. Since we synthesize animal-based proteins more easily, animal-based proteins were labeled as having a higher biological value.

As a result animal-based proteins were labeled as being "high-quality" proteins and were given a "Class A"–protein classification. Plant-based proteins were given a "Class B" classification, and over time, this led to plant-based protein being overlooked and forgotten. This led to vegans and vegetarians being asked, "Where do you get your protein?

The consumption of animal-based protein became entrenched in the American social paradigm from that time forward and was associated with one having better health.

More recently, Frances Moore Lappe, author of the popular 1971 book *Diet for a Small Planet*, promoted eating a vegetarian diet to combat world hunger, but she was concerned the diet wouldn't supply the variety and quantity of amino acids needed to support healthy living. Her concern reinforced the idea that plant-based protein was "inferior" to animal-based protein, but weakness could be addressed by "food combining" She concluded that vegetarians could be healthy only if they ate foods in particular combinations to supply all the essential amino acids needed.

Lappe reversed her views, stating, "In 1971 I stressed protein complementarity because I assumed that the only way to get enough protein…was to create a protein as usable by the body as animal protein. In combating the myth that meat is the only way to get high-quality protein, I reinforced another myth. I gave the impression that in order to get enough protein without meat, considerable care was needed in choosing foods. Actually, it is much easier than I thought…If people are getting enough calories, they are virtually certain of getting enough protein."[10]

The idea of food combining is still around today, even though it was proven scientifically to not be true. Though Lappe changed her views about food combining in her later editions of *Diet for a Small Planet*, the damage had already been done because proponents of the consumption of animal-based protein used her position to reinforce the superiority of animal-based protein. It was firmly etched in the minds of the majority of people that animal protein was the king of nutrients and that we needed to eat a lot of it to be healthy and strong.

Organizations like the American Dietetic Association also had to reverse their views of "food combing" and the inferiority of plant-based protein. "Plant sources of protein alone can provide adequate amounts of the essential and nonessential amino acids…Conscious combining of these foods within a given meal, as a complementary protein dictum suggests, is unnecessary."[11, 12] The World Health Organization (WHO) also changed its position and concluded that "few natural diets provide insufficient amounts of indispensable amino acids," as long as the diet contained enough calories. The WHO recommended people eat fifty grams of protein per 2,200 calories.[13] Even with these major organizations changing their position on the consumption of animal-based protein being superior, the thought of its superiority is still strong, and plant-based protein is an afterthought.

Animal-based protein still remains king, even after numerous studies have shown an overconsumption of animal-based proteins supports cancer development. Dr. Colin Campbell's studies showed there was a sharp increase in cancer development as animal-based protein consumption went from 10 percent to 20 percent of the diet.[14] The same relationship was not found between cancer development and plant-based protein. "By contrast, the amino acid compositions of plant proteins—always a bit of a mismatch with ours—are also less efficient at promoting unwanted growth. However, scientists were not able to intuit this relationship between protein and disease."[15]

These types of studies that showed that plant-based proteins are suitable and preferable in supporting growth and controlling cancer development made scientists rethink their early conclusions that animal-based proteins were superior to plant-based proteins. Even though scientists and nutrition organizations reversed their positions on animal-based proteins, the consumption and promotion of animal-based protein remained firmly embedded in the Western diet. The meat industry does a great job of self-preservation and promoting the consumption of animal-based foods. Science has shown that consumption more than 10 percent of animal-based protein in the diet supports cancer development, and it is clear people eating a Western diet are consuming more than that.

CHAPTER 3:

ANIMAL-BASED PROTEIN AND CANCER DEVELOPMENT

It appears there is a natural God/The Source/Nature pattern that dictates how much protein we need to sustain homeostasis. That magic number appears to be 10 percent of the diet. Dr. Campbell was a proponent of the consumption of animal-based protein in addressing malnutrition and supporting health. In the midst of his studies on protein, Dr. Campbell was confronted with evidence that supported the notion that protein consumption or excessive protein consumption as being detrimental to healthy living.

Dr. Campbell first was confronted with the results of a study of Filipino children who ate the most protein that suggested they tended to have higher rates of liver cancer. The study gave Dr. Campbell the impression that diets high in protein might be associated with liver cancer.[16] The work of researchers Madhavan and Gopalan reinforced this impression. They hypothesized that a diet low in protein would likely lead to the development of liver cancer. Their hypothesis reinforced the earlier conclusion that protein consumption was primary in supporting health. The results weren't what the researchers thought they would be.

In their study, rats were given the carcinogen aflatoxin, and some of the rats were fed diets that consisted of 20 percent protein, while the other rats were fed diets consisting of 5 percent protein. The carcinogen aflatoxin caused the mutation of healthy cells into cancerous cells, but it needed an agent to start and support the process. Animal-based protein was the agent. All the rats fed the 20 percent protein diet developed liver cancer, and none of the rats fed the 5 percent protein diet developed liver cancer.[17]

The results of the study of the Filipino children and the Madhavan and Gopalan study led Dr. Campbell and his team to perform their studies to determine protein's effect on the development of liver cancer.

Dr. Campbell used casein as his protein of choice. Casein is the main protein in milk and cheese and is also found in processed meats like hot dogs and hamburgers. The rats in his study were exposed to a carcinogen and were divided in groups that were fed 5 percent, 12 percent, and 20 percent protein diets.[18]

The normal lifespan of the rats was one hundred weeks. All the rats that were fed a 20 percent protein diet developed severe tumors and were dead well within the one hundred weeks. All the rats fed the 5 percent protein diet remained healthy within the one hundred weeks. Tumor formation was shut down when rats were switched from the 20 percent protein diet to the 5 percent protein diet at forty weeks. There was minimal tumor initiation in rats that were fed the 12 percent protein diet. Tumor development escalated severely as the percentage rose to 20 percent.

Through evaluating his studies, Dr. Campbell indicated a diet should consist of no more than 10 percent animal-based protein to minimize the risk of developing cancer. Though the studies were done with rats, rats require around the same amount of protein as humans require. People take carcinogens into their bodies on a regular basis because carcinogens are present in the air, water, and food we eat, through pollution and chemical contamination. Pollution and chemical contamination (carcinogens) alter the natural balance and composition of the environment, which sets the stage for cell mutation. Consumption of animal-based protein above 10 percent of total daily calories eaten in combination with the carcinogens already present in the environment overtaxes the body's natural defense systems that allow it to remove the carcinogens.

In contrast, Dr. Campbell's studies showed soy- and wheat-plant-based protein consumption, even up to 20 percent of the daily calories eaten, did not support cancer development. Though our bodies can compensate for the consumption of animal-based protein up to 10 percent of total daily calories eaten, it appeared that plant-based protein worked best with the natural patterns and structure of the body.

CHAPTER 4:

THE PROCESS OF CANCER DEVELOPMENT

Viruses, excessive radiation from sunlight, radiation from radioactive materials, family history or genetics, nutritional imbalances, chemical carcinogens, and possibly stress all contribute to the development of cancer. The ecosystem of God/The Source/Nature protects us from the radiation of the sunlight through the earth's protective ozone layer. The products and pollution that industry make erode the natural balance of the ecosystem, and we are now offered less protection against UV radiation from the sun.

God/The Source/Nature offers us protection against harmful viruses that also develop in the ecosystem—through the plant life it provides us for nourishment and healing. Plants protect themselves from viruses, bacteria, and other harmful substances with their phytonutrients.[19] People are provided natural protection against natural causes of cancer, but human-made causes are problematic for the body to address because they exist outside the normal development and patterns of life. The radiation and pollution we introduce into the environment and the unnatural and foreign chemicals we consume in processed foods and processed medicines greatly challenge homeostasis in the body. This causes mental and physical stresses that adversely affect our biology and genes.

Though there are multiple agents that can cause cancer, many believe the chemicals that pollute our environment and that are used in the harvesting, packaging, and processing of our food are the chief causes of cancer. Regardless of the agent, cancer development happens in the same way and is studied in three stages: initiation, promotion, and progression. Since environmental and food chemicals are believed to be the primary cause of cancer, I refer to chemicals as the agent within the three stages of cancer development.

Chemicals are thought to act primarily in the initiation stage, and these cancer-initiating chemicals are called carcinogens. The initiation stage involves the initial attachment of chemicals to cells. Once you consume, breathe in, or touch these carcinogens, they enter the body and make their way to the bloodstream. Most of the carcinogens are fat-soluble, and they seek to store themselves in fat cells. The liver produces enzymes that convert the carcinogens into water-soluble molecules called metabolites that are more easily removed from the body.

Unfortunately, at times, small amounts of carcinogens escape the full conversion process and end up being turned into highly destructive metabolites that attack DNA, RNA, and proteins.[20] Though some carcinogens are able to attack DNA, RNA, and proteins, the body is very resilient; it is able to repair most of the damage. Between 99 and 99.9 percent of the affected cells get repaired. Mutation occurs when the unrepaired cells replicate. This mutation within the initiation stage happens quickly and can occur within days. Under the right conditions, the body is able to halt the replication of mutated cells, as Dr. Campbell's study showed.[21]

Promotion is the second stage of cancer development, where mutated cells replicate to form substantial mass. Promotion can take many years to complete. Progression is the final stage where masses grow into large tumors and are able to spread from the primary site to another area of the body. This invasiveness is called metastasis and can happen in a short period.

Cancer development can be controlled under the right conditions. Dr. Campbell showed in his studies there was a push-pull process at play that is controlled by the amount of promoters and antipromoters present.[22] When more promoters were present and active, the tendency was toward cancer development. When more antipromoters were present, the tendency was toward regression. Antipromoters can be used to keep cancer in a stable state of regression, even when mutated cells remain in the body. In the case of Dr. Campbell's rat studies, the addition of animal-based protein was a promoter, and the removal of animal-based protein was an antipromoter. Nutritional imbalances also serve as promoters, while balanced nutrition serves as an antipromoter.

Many nutrients above or below their optimal levels have been shown to promote or stop cancer development. Dr. Campbell explained that in his experiments, diet higher in fat tended to increase the development of early pancreatic-cancer clusters, and human studies have shown that high-fat diets were associated with a higher risk for pancreatic cancer. Dr. Campbell and his colleagues noted in their studies that as consumption of antioxidant carotenoids (phytonutrients) increased, liver cancer decreased. As carotenoid consumption decreased, liver cancer increased.[23]

As we move away from natural, healing diets that are high in nutrient- and phytonutrient-containing plant-based life provided by God/The Source/Nature to diets that are high in animal-based protein and chemically laden processed foods, we set up an environment that is conducive to the development of cancer.

Though carcinogens can alter DNA and give rise to harmful mutated cells, mutated cells do not have the last word in determining whether they turn into cancerous tumors. Nutrition controls the expression and replication of mutated cells. Nutrition controls the promotion stage and perhaps even the progression stage of cancer development.

CHAPTER 5:

MEAT-CENTERED DIETS ARE HARMFUL TO ANIMALS AND PEOPLE

The US meat industry grows and kills nearly ten billion animals a year for food consumption.[24] That is around thirty-one times the US population. Factory-farming methods were designed to make it possible to raise so many animals for food consumption at the expense of animals. "The factory-farming industry strives to maximize output while minimizing costs—always at the animals' expenses. The giant corporations that run most factory farms have found that they can make more money by cramming animals into tiny spaces, even though many of the animals get sick and some die."[25]

I have to be optimistic and agree with Paul McCartney's statement in his video: "If slaughter houses had glass walls, everyone would be vegetarian."[26] It is evident in nature there is a natural food chain or feeding hierarchy. Some animals feed on plants, and some animals feed on the animals that feed on plants. The difference between the natural process and pattern of life and the factory-farming method is the natural process allows the animals to grow healthily and to develop bonds with each other. They have feelings and experience joy as well as pain. The factory-farming method only sees them as things and is not concerned about the animals' welfare at any point of their lives.

Some will overlook the atrocities of factory farming because it may be easy to internalize the outcome that animals still end up on the dinner plate, whether through a natural process or not. It is easy to ignore the pain of factory-farmed animals unless you are standing at the factory's glass wall, looking in.

Cows, chickens, turkeys, and other animals are crammed into small areas to maximize the use of space. Chickens and turkeys are crammed into small spaces by the tens of thousands and live in their own feces. Animals are deprived of exercise and are fed large amounts of feed to make them to grow bigger and fatter and to produce more eggs or milk. Animals are genetically modified and are also fed growth hormones to make them grow at an unnatural rate and to an unnatural size. Many of the animals would die from disease because of the conditions they live in, but they are kept alive by being fed large amounts of antibiotics.

Animals are only being grown to be killed for their meat and only know lives full of suffering. Not only do the confined, unsanitary spaces and lack of exercise encourage the development of disease, their diets also contribute to it. Cattle's natural food stock is grass, and their genetics and biology work best with it. Now factory-farming methods use corn, soy, and hay to feed cows instead of letting them roam and graze on grass. The factory-farming method purposely switched the diet of cattle to mostly grain instead of grass to fatten up the cattle for consumption. Though corn, soy, and hay are not part of their natural diet, these food stocks are much better than what cattle are fed when these food stocks run out.

Factory farmers have had to rely on some really suspect food stocks when corn, soy, and hay have become unavailable. During times when there is a shortage of corn, soy, and hay—and also as a way to keep costs down—cattle farmers have relied on feeding their cattle candy.[27, 28] Cattle have been fed gummy bears, cookies, chocolate, fruit loops, and a whole list of other candies. These processed junk foods contain harmful substances like high-fructose corn syrup, MSG, hydrogenated oils, pesticides, herbicides, insecticides, acrylamides, artificial flavorings, artificial colorings, and artificial sweeteners like aspartame.[29, 30, 31, 32] These chemically laden processed foods are harmful to the health of cattle, just as they are harmful to the health of humans.

Factory farmers have also resorted to feeding cattle sawdust. Cattle farmers have the nerve to promote it as healthy.[33, 34] Sawdust is made largely of cellulose, which is a carbohydrate, so factory farmers will argue it is good for the cattle. Unfortunately, sawdust is bound together by a compound called lignin that makes it hard to digest. Nitric acid, a highly corrosive mineral acid that is used as a precursor in the manufacturing of explosives, is used to strip the lignin from the cellulose. Some of the nitric acid remains on the cellulose that is fed to cattle, which is harmful to their digestive systems and their health.

Chicken feces have been another food-stock alternative to feed to cattle. The large amount of chicken feces produced by chickens is expensive to properly dispose of. Since chicken feces contain protein, someone came up with the idea to feed cattle chicken feces as a way of killing two birds with one stone. Cattle are fed chicken feces for protein, and the cattle help to cheaply get rid of the chicken feces. Metal, glass, rocks, and other foreign objects end up mixed into the chicken feces. Pathogens like as Salmonella typhimurium, Escherichia coli, and/or Clostridium botulinum may be present in chicken feces as the result chicken carcasses being mixed in with the chicken litter.[35, 36] The chicken feces are processed to remove the debris and kill the pathogens before they are fed to cattle, but you have to think about how much care really goes into the process when cattle are treated so horrifically in the first place.

Cattle have also been fed limestone to supplement calcium and have been fed crab, shrimp, and fish guts because they are protein sources. Though cows do eat this food that is given to them, guts are not part of their natural diet. Just like humans, cattle can eat a wide variety of foods, but it doesn't mean that the foods are good for them. Imagine what is happening to their digestive systems.

All of the interference with the cattle's natural patterns of daily life activities and eating habits has its repercussions. Factory-farming methods cause cattle to develop a wide range of diseases at a higher rate, and great amounts of antibiotics have to be administered to cattle in order to keep them alive.

Milder strains of E. coli have always been present in the stomachs of cattle, but their change to an unnatural grain diet is associated with an overall increase in total populations of E. coli, including the pathogenic bacteria E. coli strain O157:H7.[37] "Most of the microbes that reside in the gut of a cow and find their way into our food get killed off by the strong acids in our stomachs, since they evolved to live in the neutral pH environment of the rumen. But the rumen of a corn-fed feedlot steer is nearly as acidic as our own stomachs, and in this new, human-made environment, new acid-resistant strains of E. coli, of which O157:H7 is one, have evolved."[38, 39]

Methicillin-resistant Staphylococcus aureus (MRSA) infections are on the rise and factory-farmed animals are a likely reason. Initially MRSA was thought to spread only from humans to humans and was a common hospital-acquired infection. Now MRSA is also being spread from animals to humans.[40] There hasn't been much research done in the United States, but recent studies in Europe have demonstrated a strong causal link between MRSA and pig farming.[41] Animals are becoming increasingly infected with MRSA, and the bacteria are increasingly passed on to humans through contact and consumption. MRSA is also resistant to antibiotics, which can make it difficult to treat.

Campylobacter and salmonella proliferation is on the rise due to unsanitary factory-farming methods. Over 1.3 million Americans are estimated to contract the foodborne, infectious intestinal disease yearly.[42] The disease can cause abdominal pain, diarrhea, fever, nausea, and, sometimes, temporary paralysis. Campylobacter is becoming increasingly drug resistant, and its drug resistance has increased from 13 percent in 1997 to almost 25 percent in 2011.[43]

A 2010 study by Consumer Reports showed that 62 percent of chicken sold in supermarkets is contaminated with campylobacter.[44] Fourteen percent of chickens were contaminated with salmonella.

Salmonella also causes pain, diarrhea, fever, and nausea, along with headaches and vomiting.

Factory-farming methods are responsible for the development of bovine spongiform encephalopathy (BSE), also referred to as mad cow disease. The disease is the result of feeding cattle food that contains parts of butchered cattle.

Many people will still not develop a connection or empathy with cattle and other animals that are treated inhumanely because they are animals, and the people feel the animals are here to be used by the dominant human species in whatever manner seems fit. If people can't find empathy for animals, then people need to view this as a human issue. The consumption of disease-ridden animals passes on their diseases to humans who consume their meat. The factory-farmed meat consumed today has far more harmful effects on the body than the naturally raised animals of a generation ago.

Great damage is being inflicted on the human body from the consumption of disease-ridden meat. People are being flooded with diseases from these animal products, and many are not even aware of the danger. Many have come to accept the rate at which human beings are being afflicted by disease as being normal, and it is not. Not only are diseases associated with factory-farming methods proliferating, super-diseases or superbugs are developing that are either immune or are becoming immune to the antibiotics given to animals to keep them alive. This means that when people consume meat that contains these superbugs, antibiotics will have less to no effect in killing the superbugs.

Dr. Greger wrote in a research article, "Homo sapiens have dramatically altered the ecological landscape in which other species and their pathogens must function."[45] Mankind has developed industry that has altered the natural pattern of life established by God/The Source/Nature. This has had the consequence of throwing off the balance of life and has allowed disease to proliferate beyond what the natural patterns had established.

CHAPTER 6:

MEAT-CENTERED DIETS ARE DESTROYING THE EARTH'S ECOSYSTEM

Not only are meat-centered diets destroying our health and the health of animals, they are literally destroying the earth's ecosystem. This is turn will destroy life on earth. Increased meat production is directly responsible for the overuse of and great strain on energy and power systems to run factory-farming operations. Increased meat production is also directly responsible for the loss of millions of acres of tropical forest due to deforestation. The deforestation is needed to provide land for grazing animals and also to clear land to plant crops to feed factory-farmed animals. The staggering amount of grain needed to feed factory-farmed animals requires enormous amounts water to grow grain, which overtaxes the natural water supply and contributes to drought. The whole cycle contributes greatly to the amount of manufactured greenhouse gases that are released into the atmosphere and contributes to climate change.

People do not consume most of the grain crops that are grown in the United States. Seventy percent of US grain production is used to feed to livestock.[46] We still wouldn't need to produce this much excess grain for human consumption if we all stopped consuming meat and only ate a plant-based diet. The amount of crops that are needed to feed livestock grows quickly because the production of livestock keeps increasing. "The world's total meat supply was 71 million tons in 1961. In 2007, it was estimated to be 284 million tons. Per capita consumption has more than doubled over that period. (In the developing world, it rose twice as fast, doubling in the last 20 years.) World meat consumption is expected to double again by 2050, which one expert, Henning Steinfeld of the United Nations, says is resulting in a 'relentless growth in livestock production.'"[47] As the unnatural level of livestock production increases, deforestation, the production of grain, and the overuse of natural resources increase to sustain the production.

Americans represent around 5 percent of the world's total population, but the United States grows and kills around ten billion animals a year, which is around 15 percent of the world's total. This is an incredible number of animals being slaughtered every year in just the United States alone to satisfy a food craving. It is a craving because it is established that meat consumption is not necessary to support health. This overproduction of animals puts great strain on our environment, ecosystem, and the God/The Source/Nature patterns that govern life.

Five million acres of South and Central American forests are cut down every year to clear land for cattle to graze to satisfy our cravings for meat. At least one hundred animals are added to the endangered species list each year, and grazing livestock are responsible for harming around 20 percent of all endangered animals.[48] Overgrazing during the past half century damaged more than 60 percent of the world's rangelands.[49] Overgrazing has degraded as much as 85 percent of rangeland in the western United States. Thirty-five pounds of topsoil are lost in the production of one pound of grain-fed beef.[50] Cropland lost worldwide due to soil erosion is twenty-five million acres, and twenty-five million acres is due to salinization. In the United States, eleven tons of soil per acre per year is lost to soil erosion.[51]

Nitrogen-based fertilizer is used to combat soil erosion. Constantly growing crops on the same land over time depletes the nutrients in the soil. Using nitrogen-based fertilizer replenishes nutrients, which sustains crop production and also creates another problem. A lot of the nitrogen fertilizer ends up running off the land into streams, lakes, and the coastal oceans.

The nitrogen fertilizer runs off into the coastal oceans and feeds algae and increases algae growth beyond what is normal.[52] The unnatural large bodies of algae eventually die and settle into the coastline. Microbes then feed on the dead algae and consume large amounts of oxygen. Oxygen levels become low (hypoxic) or nonexistent (anoxic). All oxygen-consuming organisms in the hypoxic and anoxic areas die from suffocation, including fish. These hypoxic and anoxic are called dead zones for good reason.

Besides deforestation, endangering of animal species, and land and ocean erosion, water consumption needed to support meat production also presents a serious problem. It takes 5,000 gallons of water to produce one pound of beef, while it takes 250 gallons of water to produce one pound of bread.[53] Water consumption is becoming a big problem in the United States. A combined study[54] from NASA, Columbia University, and Cornell University predicted a megadrought to occur over the next thirty-five years in the Southwest and Great Plains areas of the United States. It will last longer and be more severe than any other droughts that have occurred in the last thousand years. The research showed that natural patterns of drought are now being amplified and extended because of the excessive use of water and greenhouse gases being released into the environment.

"Agriculture is a major user of ground and surface water in the United States, accounting for approximately 80 percent of the nation's consumptive water use and over 90 percent in many Western States."[55] Most of this water goes to grow crops to support animal production and is not for human consumption.

The fossil-energy requirements to produce livestock are staggering and contribute to greenhouse gases being released into the atmosphere. The increased greenhouse gases have a detrimental effect on climate change because greenhouse gases absorb infrared radiation from the sun and trap the heat in the atmosphere. Along with the extreme amount of water used to support meat production, rising temperatures also help to diminish the water supply. The most important greenhouses gases that affect climate change are carbon dioxide, methane, and nitrous oxide. Other gases like those found in aerosols also contribute to the buildup of greenhouse gases and climate change.

The American Journal of Clinical Nutrition estimates the average fossil-energy input for all the animal-protein production systems studied (beef, chicken, and lamb) is 25 kcal of fossil energy per 1 kcal of meat produced. The energy used is around eleven times that for crop production. 2.2 kcal of fossil energy is used to produce 1 kcal of grain.[56] The energy inputs required to feed the average vegetarian is 33 percent less than a person who is a carnivore. The energy inputs required to sustain a vegan is 50 percent less than a carnivore.[57]

The United Nations Food and Agriculture Organization estimates that livestock production generates nearly a fifth of the world's greenhouse gases, which is more than transportation produces. Japan's National Institute of Livestock and Grassland Science estimated that 2.2 pounds of beef is responsible for using the equivalent amount of energy used to light a one-hundred-watt light bulb for twenty days, and is responsible for emitting the equivalent amount of carbon dioxide the average European car emits every 155 miles.[58]

The United Nations published a report indicating agriculture, particularly meat and dairy products, accounts for 70 percent of global freshwater consumption, 38 percent of the total land use, and 14 percent of the world's manufactured greenhouse-gas emissions.[59] The 14 percent of greenhouse gases added to the environment from meat and dairy production only accounts for the direct addition of greenhouses.

Meat production is responsible for alarming rates of deforestation across the world. Deforestation is needed to clear land for grazing animals and for planting crops to feed factory-farmed animals. Deforestation accounts for 17 percent of the manufactured greenhouse-gas emissions. Energy supply accounts for 26 percent, and transport accounts for 13 percent of greenhouses made from human industry. A chunk of the percentage is involved in supplying power for meat and dairy production and for transporting meat and dairy products.

Though natural patterns of drought do exist, human intervention is definitely making them worse than they need to be. The United Nations says decreased consumption of animal products and a move toward a plant-based diet are necessary to save the world from the worst impacts of climate change.

The high consumption of meat goes against the natural order of life. It throws the life of our ecosystem out of balance. God/The Source/Nature had determined this balance, and humans were meant to live within the balance, along with all the other life on the earth. I am cautious not to say the consumption of meat goes against the natural order of life. We do see in nature that animals eat other animals. Meat-eating animals generally eat grazing animals. Since humans are at the top of the food chain and are able to digest meat, it is easy to see that humans would eat meat. The issue is that the consumption of meat on a daily basis is a modern practice.

Eating meat at one time was a luxury because people couldn't afford it, and meat was a sacrifice of money or time to attain. Eating small portions of meat, maybe once or twice a week, was more the norm in the past. Eating small amounts of meat infrequently also allowed the body to compensate for damage that meat consumption did to it. The damage done in the past was far less severe than the damage done presently by factory-farmed and processed meat, and mercury- and toxin-laden fish.

Meat is still very expensive to produce, and naturally costs more to produce than plant-based foods. We don't see the expense, though, because the government subsidizes the meat and fishing industries. This lowers meat- and fish-production costs and allows for meat and fish to be sold below cost. Our taxpayer dollars pay for this subsidy, which had to be put in place to satisfy our cravings for meat consumption. So individuals who rely heavily on meat consumption keep the demand for meat production high and keep the subsidies in place.

The high demand for meat results in deforestation, endangering wildlife species, overconsumption of energy, greenhouse gases, land erosion, sea erosion, and destructive climate change. The high demand for animal products is damaging the natural order of our ecosystem put in place by God/The Source/Nature, and without the natural order, God/The Source/Nature will stop supporting life on earth.

CHAPTER 7:

THE BUSINESS OF NUTRITION PROMOTES THE OVERCONSUMPTION OF MEAT, UNNATURAL FOOD PRODUCTS, AND VITAMIN SUPPLEMENTS

Please realize that everything is business. Though we may expect health industries to be altruistic and hold the welfare and health of people over all other agendas, they often do not. The bottom line is to make profit, and vested interests will push the limits of health claims and regulations to make a profit. The health industry influences scientific studies to support the products that it produces, and whole plant-based foods are not one of those products.

Dr. Campbell broke down the health industry down into four sectors that include the food industry, drug industry, dietary-supplement industry, and the medical-practice industry, which includes hospitals and doctors. Dr. Campbell spent a great deal of his life doing research that had been used and sometimes misused to shape public policy. Public policy is the foundation for shaping government programs, programs like MyPlate, formerly known as the food pyramid, school lunch programs, and the Women, Infants, and Children's program (WIC).

The health industry's influence on shaping public policy starts with lobbying Congress[60] to ensure most of the funding the National Institutes of Health (NIH) goes to supporting its agenda. The NIH is a US government agency that is the most influential biomedical-research agency in the world. It conducts health research and develops health policies that shape the paradigms of not only the American people, but also people of countries around the world. Since these sectors exercise economic influence over US government policy making, these sectors are able to severely influence what type of research gets done and what people think.

The health industry lobbies for research funding to go toward drug, genetics, and nutrient-supplement research and development, which allows for the development and sale of products based on the research. Little money goes into plant-based nutrition research because it is not a lucrative business, but plants are a gift from God/The Source/Nature.

On top of the unbalanced government funding that is in favor of industry interests, there is also the concern that researchers are sometimes being paid under the table to support industry agendas.

Industry lobbying and payoffs have played a direct role in animal-based foods, processed foods, and vitamin supplements dominating diets, even though science has shown them to be detrimental to health. These following examples show how industry influence drives the consumption of animal-based and processed foods.

Dr. Campbell's professional involvement in research that informed public-health policy kept him close to major events in the health sector. These events involved manipulation of nutritional data and unethical business by the health industry. The health industry's manipulation led to the promotion the consumption of animal-based foods, processed foods, and vitamin supplementation over natural plant-based foods.

The Dietary Guidelines Committee and Food and Nutrition Board of National Academy of Sciences are two organizations that played a large part in determining US nutritional policy. The Dietary Guidelines Committee developed the food pyramid, which is now known as MyPlate.[61] This food pyramid was highly influential in reinforcing in the paradigms of Americans about the foods that were necessary to support health, and milk and meat were high on its list. This happened because the Department of Agriculture had strong ties to the livestock industry, and it also basically ran the Dietary Guidelines Committee that produces the food pyramid. There has been constant controversy surrounding the food pyramid report because of concerns about bias from the Department of Agriculture toward animal-based foods over plant-based foods.

The committee that had been putting together the recommendations for the food pyramid had been operating unethically and with conflict of interests concerning the public's health. A court order had to be issued to bring the conflict of interest to light. The committee was forced by court order to reveal their business associations, and six of the eleven members were found to have private-sector associations with the dairy industry.[62] The court also found that the chairperson of the committee had taken more than the maximum amount of money from the private sector that was allowed without making it public record. Basically, those members of the committee had financial reasons to have a bias for animal-based foods for over plant-based foods. "Having advisors tied to the meat or dairy industries is as inappropriate as letting tobacco companies decide our standards for air quality," said PCRM president Neal D. Barnard, MD.

The chairperson of the Dietary Guidelines Committee, who had ties to the dairy industry, also happened to be the chairperson of the Food and Nutrition Board (FNB) in 2002. The board at that time received 49 percent of their funding from industry sources, which was something that was unheard of before that. The ties to industry represented a conflict of interest. This was very disturbing because the Food and Nutrition Board's 2002 report veered away from established levels of nutrient consumption in favor of increased protein, fat, and processed-carbohydrate consumption.[63]

The Food and Nutrition Board meets every five years and sets the recommended daily allowances (RDAs) for the nutrients we should consume. The RDA for protein before the release of the report was 10 percent of the total calories consumed. Recommendations for protein consumption were established based on scientific calculations of the body's use of protein. The first recommendations were established as the Estimated Average Requirement (EAR), which was formerly known as the Minimum Daily Requirement (MDR).[64] The EAR for protein was set at 4–5 percent of total daily calories. Since the EAR was the average that meant that 50 percent of the population actually needed less than 4–5 percent of total calories to come from protein, while 50 percent of the population needed more.

The RDA addressed this issue. The RDA added two standard deviations to the EAR, which meant the majority of people consuming the RDA were consuming much more protein than needed. The RDA raised protein consumption from 4–5 percent of total daily calories to 10 percent of daily calories. This was the maximum amount of protein needed to support homeostasis in the body, and scientific research had shown the consumption of animal-based protein above the amount actually supported the development of disease.

From the release of the report forward, the recommended allowance for protein skyrocketed from 10 percent to 35 percent[65] of daily calories, which was promoted to reduce the risk of chronic disease. The recommendation was made though science showed animal-based protein consumption above 10 percent of total calories was detrimental to health.

The board raised the RDA for fat from 30 percent to 35 percent and recommended children could consume fat up to 40 percent of total calories eaten. Dr. Campbell was part of a committee that produced the National Academy of Sciences' Diet and Nutrition Report in 1982.[66] The report recommended the reduction of the consumption of fat from the average 38–40 percent down to 30 percent of total daily calories to reduce the risk of cancer. This report helped set the RDA for fat. The committee had data to justify lowering their recommendation even further, debated if the percentage was low enough to reduce the risk of developing cancer, but decided to stay at 30 percent of total daily calories. Raising the RDA for fat went against previous studies and appeared to be solely the result the FNB's association with industry.

The FNB's 2012 report also concluded that 25 percent of total calories could come from processed carbohydrates, which included additive sugar, candy, pastries, and cakes. Looking at these combined recommendations, it is clear to see that there was a bias toward industry and the products it developed over whole, plant-based foods. These percentages totally excluded the consumption of plant-based foods and the natural vitamins, minerals, and phytonutrients they provided. Industry products in the form of vitamin supplements, though, could easily address the lack of nutrient consumption, which likely would happen as a result of following the updated of recommendations. There are science-based issues with the use of vitamin supplements, though.

In the same Diet and Nutrition Report in 1982, Dr. Campbell and his committee concluded based on research that a strong focus should be put on the consumption of fruits, vegetables, and whole-grain foods. The studies indicated that the nutrients in these foods were protective against cancer and protective of health. The committee strongly cautioned against obtaining these nutrients from vitamin supplements and strongly urged that these nutrients be obtained through the consumption of fruits, vegetables, and whole-grain foods.

Though the focus of the report was on the nutrients in fruits, vegetables, and whole-grain foods, industry used the media to focus on and promote the use of nutrient supplements. After the release of the report, there was a boom in the supplement industry that turned it into a multimillion-dollar industry. Industry was extremely successful in misrepresenting the report's recommendation by running full-page ads in publications like *Time* magazine linking nutrient supplements with cancer prevention. Because so many people were reeled into buying supplements to combat cancer, the Federal Trade Commission had to get involved and held hearings over the next three years from the report's release to refute the claims that the use of nutrient supplements was protective against cancer.[67]

Even though Dr. Campbell and the committee cautioned about the focus on nutrient supplements, the National Cancer Institute spent hundreds of millions of dollars on randomized clinical trials over the next twenty years and still struggled to find evidence that nutrient supplements could prevent cancer. The use of nutrient supplements did show beneficial effects in the short run, if you had a proven deficiency. In the long run, the use of nutrient supplements was ineffective in supporting healthy, and in some cases they were detrimental to health.[68, 69, 70]

These examples show why it is difficult to know how to approach proper nutrition. Industry has been able to manipulate the research process and promote foods and products that science has shown to not be in the best interest in supporting proper nutrition and health. Through lobbying Congress, industry has also been able to influence government research agencies to focus their research funding into supporting the development of health-industry products and technology. This was done at the expense of focusing funding into researching the benefits of whole, plant-based foods in supporting health and fighting disease, which science has strongly supported as being able to fight disease and to support health.

Though funding has been low for plant-based foods research, researchers have persevered through the funding obstacles and have been able to provide valuable data supporting the benefits of plant-based foods. Dr. Campbell also played in vital part in providing compelling scientific data that supported benefits of plant-based foods and a plant-based diet through his China Project study and book, *The China Study*. Though numerous scientists have published studies supporting the health benefits of plant-based foods over animal-based foods, contradictory studies and opinions based on industry-driven studies keep people confused about how to pursue healthy living.[71]

CHAPTER 8:

INSTEAD OF BEING A PART OF GOD/THE SOURCE/NATURE, WE ARE NOW APART

As a race, we have made great technological and industrial strides that have given us great command over the earth's resources. Some would say these strides have made us closer to God, and some believe we have become closer to being gods. The reality is the ease at which we gain things, as a result of many technological and industrial strides, has resulted in gluttony and the loss of connection to and appreciation of the life around us. It has slowly eroded our humanity and has made us apart from God/The Source/Nature.

Humanity as a whole is out of balance with God/The Source/Nature, which is manifested in the earth's ecosystem and the life it contains. Veering away from the consumption of the natural and life-sustaining plant-based foods that God/The Source/Nature has provided, in favor of meat- and processed-food-dominated diets, is destroying our bodies and is making illness epidemic.

Not only is this approach responsible for the destruction of the health of humans, the overconsumption of the world's resources is throwing life out of balance as a whole and is leading toward the destruction of the earth's ecosystem. Though industry's manipulation of data and people is the root of this destruction, people have to understand this only happens because people support industry's agenda by consuming and purchasing its products. People consume unnatural amounts of meat, which pushes the meat industry to keep up with the demand for its supply. This in turn has its detrimental repercussions of increasing greenhouse gases in the atmosphere to levels that support harmful climate change and the destruction of the earth's ecosystem. People are not exempt from the responsibility of caring for the earth just because the majority are not producers of these products. People are not exempt from living within the natural patterns of life that God/The Source/Nature had established.

Human beings are at the top of the chain of life on earth because of unparalleled self-awareness, and this places a great amount of responsibility on humans. This self-awareness allows humans to gain conscious understanding of the patterns that God/The Source/Nature has established within the earth's ecosystem, which allows for the manipulations of the patterns to make tools and industry. The responsibility of this self-awareness is reflected in wisdom to understand when the tools and industry manipulate the patterns to a point of harm.

An example of this involves the natural balance of greenhouse gases in the atmosphere that regulate the absorption of radiation from the sun and the temperature on earth. To satisfy the unnaturally large consumption of animal products, the meat industry cuts down life-sustaining, carbon-dioxide-absorbing, and oxygen-giving forests by the millions of acres. Along with the greenhouse gases the meat industry produces, the amount of greenhouse gases that human industry introduces into the atmosphere has thrown off the natural and protective of greenhouse gases that God/The Source/Nature had provided in the earth's ecosystem.

There is a lack of wisdom in continuing this process, because it harms the earth and all life it sustains. We must understand that even though industry has an agenda to maximize its profits at all costs, and it uses government policy and media to manipulate people into consuming its products, it is ultimately people who are responsible through their individual actions for the destruction of the natural, life-sustaining, God/The Source/Nature-given patterns of life. Many of our collective lives have now become about controlling the natural order of things instead of learning to live within them.

This ideology has permeated our eating habits and has interfered with our personal connection to God/The Source/Nature. Our bodies are constructed from the natural order of life and need to be fed natural foods to maintain their health. The basic principle is that God/The Source/Nature is all around us, and we are part of God/The Source/Nature. People and life around us are made up of a natural order of building blocks, components, and elements that produce synergy in their predesigned combinations.

Eating food that grows from the earth best supports the health of the body, which also can be viewed as temple of God/The Source/Nature.

Since God/The Source/Nature allowed people the self-awareness to understand the patterns of God/The Source/Nature in people as well as the rest of life, the bodies of people are the finite temples for the infinite knowledge of God/The Source/Nature. When we keep the temple strong through reinforcing it with natural plant foods that are derived from the natural, sustaining patterns of life, we strengthen our connection to God/The Source/Nature.

We consist of our minds and our bodies, and both of these direct our spiritual and emotional responses. The body can exist in a positive state of being that produces calmness, alertness, energy, ease, relaxedness, patience, compassion, and love. It can also exist in a negative state of being that produces agitation, frustration, anger, impatience, tiredness, and dullness of mind. Natural, plant-based life provides the mind and body with nutrients in specific combinations that help to keep it in a positive state of being called homeostasis.[72, 73]

The body is constantly working to keep all of its functions operating at peak efficiency to keep itself in a positive state. It does this by utilizing the nutrients we consume to keep cells strong and to repair damaged cells. When the body doesn't get the nutrients it requires, it has to do an internal balancing act to address the internal imbalance as best as possible. An example would be the body borrowing calcium from bones to keep the blood near a pH of 7.4.[74, 75, 76] This would weaken bones to keep the extremely important blood pH at the right level to support numerous functions in the body.

This has an adverse effect on physiological functions and one's state of being. Eating a well-balanced plant-based diet, or a diet that consists heavily of plant-based foods and excludes processed foods, supports all the functions of the body so it doesn't have to favor one function over another to stay as close to a state of homeostasis as it can. The body has a predetermined structure that is strengthened by predetermined foods, and God/The Source/Nature determined that order.

CHAPTER 9:

DR. SEBI AND THE POWER OF NATURAL PLANT-BASED FOODS

I had to take a leap of faith to adopt a plant-based diet. I had to fight against the established paradigm that promoted the consumption of animal-based products, processed foods, and vitamin supplements that supposedly addressed their vitamin deficiencies. I was encouraged by the methodology of the herbalist Dr. Sebi to take a giant leap of faith and give a plant-based diet a try.

I studied Dr. Sebi's methodology before I participated in Dr. Campbell's plant-based certificate course and before I became aware of the numerous meta-analyses of Dr. Greger, which exposed the power of natural plant-based foods.[77] I had to take a leap of faith to hurdle the seeds of doubt planted in my consciousness by the industry-driven reductionist paradigm, because I didn't have the science of Dr. Campbell and Dr. Greger that supported the benefits of plant-based foods and a plant-based diet.

The reductionist paradigm basically reinforced the notion that if science hasn't given its stamp of approval, then the idea was not worth much. The problem was there was little science being done to uncover the benefits of plant-based foods, and most of the studies done were supported by industry and promoted the consumption of animal-based foods and processed foods.

Even with the looming obstacle of the reductionist paradigm as a deterrent, the methodology and history of Dr. Sebi was so intriguing it compelled me to try a plant-based diet. I had nothing to lose. I just had to eat plant-based foods instead of animal-based foods for a while, and if I didn't like the results, I could always return to how I had been eating.

Dr. Sebi's philosophy and methodology revolved around the idea that illness began where the mucous membrane had been compromised. The Western medical point of view looked at disease as a result of being infected with a virus, bacteria, or fungus, and treatment was aimed toward killing these invaders. People constantly come in contact with viruses, bacteria, and fungi, but that doesn't mean a person necessarily had to become sick.

Sickness set in when the organisms and toxins that could cause disease in the body penetrated the mucous membrane of organs and disrupted cell function. The role of the mucous membrane was to keep the tissue it protected moist and to play a part in the immune system to produce mucus to trap and neutralize disease and toxins for their removal from the body.[78] When the mucous membrane throughout the body remained strong and intact, harmful organisms and toxins could not penetrate it and harm organs. They remained in the bloodstream where they were more easily targeted by the immune system and removed from the body.

The Western philosophy and methodology focused on killing the offending organisms and neutralizing toxins but did not address the underlying issue of the organ's weakened mucous membrane. This methodology allowed for the cycle of illness to continue to exist. People constantly encountered disease and toxins, but that didn't mean people had to become sick. A strong immune system protected against disease and toxins, and a strong, protective, and healthy mucous membrane was part of that immune system.

Dr. Sebi's philosophy, which was rooted in traditional medicine and herbalism, revolved around the concept that an acidic environment and excess mucus compromised the mucous membrane and therefore compromised the immune system. This allowed disease that would normally have been flushed out of the body to take a foothold and overwhelm organ and cell function.

Following this train of thought, if the mucous membrane in the lungs were compromised, the resulting illness would be pneumonia. A compromised mucous membrane in the bronchial tubes would result in bronchitis. In the pancreas, the result would be diabetes. In the joints, the result would be arthritis. The consumption of dairy products and acidic foods, which consists of cow's milk, meat, and processed foods, caused the mucous membrane to become compromised.

The body would respond to the consumption of milk and the toxins it contained with increased mucous production and inflammatory processes to combat the perceived threat. Casein, a protein in milk, had been previously linked to an increased risk of developing cancer.[79] Casein consumption had also been implicated in the overproduction of mucus in the gut and respiratory glands, which also compromised the integrity of the mucous membrane and the organs it was protecting.[80, 81]

Heavy and continuous consumption of meat and processed foods also compromised the mucous membrane because of the chronic acidic environment they developed in the body. This consumption weakened the protective mucous membrane of organs over time. Disease thrived in an acidic environment, while it also shut down the immune system. Dr. Marcial-Vega, a renowned oncologist trained at Johns Hopkins University, gave a perfect example of this.[82, 83] Through his studies, he realized that an acidic environment wreaked havoc on the immune system and aided in the proliferation of disease.

Dr. Marcial-Vega examined the blood of his cancer patients and found red blood cells lost hemoglobin, became anemic, and clumped together to protect themselves against the acidic environment of his patients. This interfered with proper oxygenation of red blood cells and the delivery of oxygen to organs to support cell function. The acidic environment also paralyzed white blood cells, which allowed for uric acid and cholesterol to build up and for harmful organisms and toxins to go unchecked.

Dr. Marcial-Vega was able to raise his patient's pH level to 7.4 simply by having them drink goji-berry juice. He used goji-berry juice at the time because he found it was the quickest natural way to turn the acidic environment of his patient's bodies into a slightly alkaline environment. The change helped to protect and strengthen their immune systems, which included their bodies' mucous membranes. The change to an alkaline environment allowed the red blood cells to separate and become properly oxygenated. This allowed for the proper and timely delivery of oxygen and nutrients to organs to support healthy cell function. White blood cells woke up from their dormant state and were able to seek and neutralize built-up uric acid, cholesterol, and harmful organisms.

Dr. Marcial-Vega's patients experienced the following while participating in the goji-berry experiment:

- Ninety percent of his patients had a reversal of acidity to alkalinity.
- Eighty-five percent of his obese patients experienced significant weight reduction with an increase in lean body mass (no loss of muscle).
- Eighty percent maintained constant levels of hemoglobin, platelets, and white blood cells. That was significant considering cancer patients undergoing cancer treatment usually experience an 80–100 percent drop in these blood levels.
- Ninety percent of his patients had a reversal of acidity to alkalinity.
- Eighty-five percent of his obese patients experienced significant weight reduction with an increase in lean body mass (no loss of muscle).
- Eighty percent maintained constant levels of hemoglobin, platelets, and white blood cells. That was significant considering cancer patients undergoing cancer treatment usually experience an 80–100 percent drop in these blood levels.

- Eighty percent of his patients with high blood pressure experienced a drop in their blood pressure. Fifty percent had to decrease or eliminate their high-blood-pressure medication.
- Seventy-five percent of all his patients experienced an increase in libido.
- Sixty-seven percent of his patients with high cholesterol experienced a minimum drop of points in four weeks.
- Sixty-four percent of his diabetic patients experienced a decrease in blood-sugar levels.

Dr. Sebi's methodology focused on the reduction of the consumption of milk and acidic foods to eliminate a mucus-ridden acidic environment, in order to protect the immune system's mucous-membrane layer. The reduction of an acidic environment was achieved through consumption of natural alkaline foods in the form of natural plant-based life. Dr. Marcial-Vega's experiment supported the premise that an acidic environment compromised the immune system and supported the proliferation of disease. His treatment also supported the notion that alkaline foods were supportive of the immune system and that they created an environment that was inhospitable to disease.

CHAPTER 10:

UNDERSTANDING THE ROLE OF PH IN THE BODY

The body works diligently to keep the blood and fluids at a slightly alkaline state near a pH of 7.4 to support homeostasis and health. The symbol *pH* stands for "potential hydrogen" and is the ability of molecules to attract hydrogen ions. The scale for the pH measurement ranges from 0 to 14, and 0 represents the highest acidic level and 14 represents the highest alkaline level. When the body doesn't get enough alkaline material to maintain a pH of 7.4, it will cause an adverse reaction to try to maintain homeostasis. For example, the body will leach calcium from bones, at the expense of bones, to maintain the proper pH in the blood, fluids, and cells.[84, 85, 86] This leaching can lead to the development of osteoporosis and result in a reduction of bone density and bone fractures.

Too many hydrogen ions floating around the bloodstream would make the blood acidic and would interfere with the proper oxygenation in the body. The body uses oxygen to release energy from molecules so organs can use the energy to perform their functions. Without the required energy, organ function becomes compromised, resulting in lethargy and illness. An acidic environment wreaks havoc on the immune system's white blood cells and causes them to go into a dormant state. This allows bacteria, viruses, and fungi to proliferate, attack weakened organs, and interfere with normal and health bodily functions.

Homeostasis and health is supported by this simple and natural pattern. Plant-based foods are loaded with natural sources of vitamins, minerals, phytonutrients, and carbohydrates. They also contain fat and protein but usually in smaller concentrations. Plants derive their nutrients from elements they absorb from the earth. Each type of plant is made up of different ratios and combinations of nutrients, depending on its natural genetic makeup.

Plants' nutrient makeups and synergies of nutrients help them to grow strong and vibrant, while plants' phytonutrients protect them against environmental pathogens. Plants absorb the sun's energy through the process of photosynthesis and converts it into physical forms of energy it uses for growth and chemical processes. Natural patterns of element and compounds develop in balance and in relation to the earth and sun's patterns of energy.

People consume the plants and absorb their natural balance of elements, compounds, and energy that are manifested in their vitamins, minerals, phytonutrients, carbohydrates, fats, and proteins. As with plants, the human body is derived from these same elements and compounds that form in response to the earth and the sun's patterns of energy. When people consume plant life, they are consuming elements and compounds that are of the same or are similar in makeup to what is in the body.

The body works to maintain a pH of 7.4 and natural non-hybrid-plant-based foods naturally provide nutrients that support this alkalinity level, while animal-based foods do not. Plant-based life contains both acidic and alkaline compounds, but their balance tends to fall on the slightly alkaline side and supports a pH of 7.4.

The body needs certain combinations of these alkalinity-promoting nutrients to support balance and homeostasis. Plant-based foods naturally provide nutrients in these combinations, but vitamin supplementation does not. Numerous studies have shown that vitamin supplementation increased mortality,[87, 88] while the nutrients in plant-based foods supported life.

A well-balanced, whole-food, plant-based diet is naturally high in vitamins, minerals, and phytonutrients to support bodily functions. It is also high in natural carbohydrates that the body burns quickly for quick access to energy. Natural carbohydrates are the body's primary fuel source. A whole-food, plant-based diet is also naturally low in fat and protein and is naturally compromised of around 80 percent carbohydrates, 10 percent fat, and 10 percent protein. God/The Source/Nature naturally provides this balance.

This balanced is comprised mostly of quickly burning carbohydrate fuel to support an energetic, work-producing body. It supplies the small amount of fat needed to support bodily functions, such as providing insulation for organs, storage of fat-soluble vitamins, and supporting brain function, growth, and cell functions.[89, 90] It also supplies the small amount of protein needed to support antibody and enzyme production, transport of components, building and maintenance of cells, and transmittal of messages throughout the body.[91] The 10 percent protein provided by whole-food, plant-based diets fully supported the RDA of 10 percent for protein, which was the maximum amount of protein needed by the body up until the Food and Nutrition Board's industry-influenced 2002 recommendation changed.

CHAPTER 11:

OVERCOMING DOUBT BEFORE ADOPTING A PLANT-BASED DIET

My personal dietary and health journey took a tremendous turn because of the frustration a lingering cold caused me. I had always suffered from sinus and chest congestion, and I would research ways of dealing with the congestion. My gradual removal of meat from my diet over many years of my life helped a lot with controlling my congestion, but there was still much room for improvement. Through health forums I interacted with, I came upon information about an herbalist named Dr. Sebi who had supposedly cured people of supposedly incurable diseases through the use of "African Bio-mineral Balance" plant-based tonics.

I was given a video claiming he cured an entertainer named Lisa Nicole Lopes ("Left Eye Lopes") of herpes. I was very skeptical of this claim. I decided to research Dr. Sebi and found that he and his USHA Research Institute claimed to be able to reverse AIDS, sickle-cell anemia, lupus, diabetes, arthritis, cancers, leukemia, herpes, epilepsy, fibroid tumors, and a host of other diseases. These claims would result in his labeling by some as a quack.

My research revealed that in 1988, Attorney General Robert Abrams took the herbalist Dr. Sebi to court for an advertisement he placed in a newspaper claiming that he cured AIDS and other diseases. The attorney general brought charges against Dr. Sebi for practicing medicine without a license and for making audacious claims about curing incurable diseases. The end result was Dr. Sebi beat the case.[92, 93] Dr. Sebi was required to present nine patients he had supposedly cured, and they had to present medical records from accredited medical institutions showing the diseases they had prior to receiving treatment from Dr. Sebi's USHA Institute. Seventy-seven patients appeared in court to support him with their medical records, and he was able to beat the case against him. The state allowed Dr. Sebi to continue his work in reversing disease using his "African Bio-mineral Balance" plant-based tonics.

Even though the claims he made were incredible, the evidence that backed his claims and the reasoning of his methodology made me give a plant-based diet a try. I felt that with the incredible claims he made, at a minimum his methodology should be able to clear up my lifelong congestion issues. I had been fighting a lingering cold for weeks during the winter when I decided to try a plant-based diet. Within one week, my congestion issues had gone away, and in the four years since I adopted a plant-based diet, I haven't had any congestion issues, such as pneumonia and other issues that have plagued me, including the flu, chest congestion, sinus congestion, and my persistent and pesky colds. I haven't had a headache, my body heals much faster from injury, and my weight dropped from the 180s to a lightest 151 pounds. I can think more clearly now, my energy is high all day, and I am able to sleep well during the night.

CHAPTER 12:

MY PATH BEFORE THE PLANT-BASED DIET

I was a pescatarian for several years before I adopted a plant-based diet, and I was very content with just eating fish and a little bit of dairy. Throughout the years of my life, I gradually removed pork, beef, and poultry from my diet and settled on only eating fish and a little bit of dairy. I was never particularly fond of milk and yogurt, so most of the dairy I ate was cheese and ice cream. I thought eating this way would categorize me as a vegetarian, but I realized that was an incorrect label.

A Rastafarian who ran a health-food store I frequented informed me that I wasn't a vegetarian. He told me the fish I ate was more of a vegetarian than I was. He let me know that there was another step I needed to take before I could be considered a vegetarian, and that step involved me giving up eating fish. I was definitely on a path of finding the healthiest foods to eat, but I wasn't ready to give up eating fish, and I never thought I would be ready. I would eat as healthy as I could, but I couldn't see myself giving up eating fish.

I didn't think I could become much healthier than I was at the time by giving up fish. I loved eating fish, and I ate it almost every day. I loved my ackee and saltfish, brown-stew kingfish, brown-stew red snapper, and fried tilapia. I felt good about where my food journey had taken me up to that point. I say journey because I wasn't always a pescatarian, and it was a journey getting to there. I didn't have a particular destination for where I wanted my diet to lead me. It was just something that happened, or something I was led to. I used to eat pork, beef, chicken, turkey, and fish, though I didn't eat shellfish. Pork was the first thing I removed from my diet.

I stopped eating pork when I was thirteen, and I am presently forty-seven. I used to pig out on ham sandwiches, and my body started to reject them. I stared to get nauseous just from the smell of ham, and it turns out that was a very good thing. Today, the factory-farming process makes meat consumption very harmful, but pork's very nature makes its consumption very harmful, even without the factory-farming process.

Pork contains tapeworms called cysticerci that invade the brain and damage the central nervous system. The disease is called neurocysticercosis, and it is the number-one cause of epilepsy in the world.[94, 95] This parasitic disease was more common is developing countries, but now this brain invasion has become a problem in the United States in the last thirty years.

Cysticersi create cavities in the brain where they can grow from two to seven meters (twenty-three feet) in length while feeding off brain tissue. These parasites also infect muscles and other tissue throughout the body. Cysticersi can live up to twenty-five years and cause a wide variety of problems, ranging from seizures, aneurysms, brain tumors, dementia, and depression to muscle pain and weakness.

I started studying different religions and philosophies heavily when I was thirteen, including Christianity, Judaism, Islam, Buddhism, Taoism, and Hinduism. One thing I had taken away from my studies was the importance of avoiding gluttony and avoiding putting things into my body that would weaken it. I also learned that people were elevated over all of creation because of people's conscious connection to God/The Source/Nature.

The body was the temple for that elevated consciousness and connection to God/The Source/Nature. People's consciousness was a gift that let them understand how God/The Source/Nature establishes the beautiful natural patterns. The body had to be kept strong, though, through eating good, healthy foods to keep the connection to God/The Source/Nature strong. A weakened body interfered with a positive emotional and mental state of being that is ultimately achieved through aligning with the natural patterns of God/The Source/Nature. Even though it took me a long time to get to where I am today, the seed was planted and grew.

The insight I gained and my pork-induced sickness made me completely give up pork. I then removed beef from my diet when I was sixteen. I suffered from excruciating migraine headaches and when I gave up eating beef, my migraine headaches went away. My headaches were so bad that I would often load up on aspirin or some other headache-relieving medicine and cry from the pain until I was able to escape it by falling asleep. Studies show the consumption of meat triggers migraines in some people,[96] and it appears that beef was my trigger.

Removing pork and beef from my diet was good for my overall health, but I still had some health issues. During my late twenties to early thirties, my weight went up to nearly two hundred pounds, though I had removed pork and beef from my diet. Weighing two hundred pounds was a lot for me because I was only five feet nine inches tall. My weight didn't bother me because it was equally distributed over my entire body, and I thought my weight gain was a natural part of growing older. My energy level was horrible, though, and I also associated that with the normal process of getting older.

I still suffered from periodic nasal and chest congestion from the flu or cold. I'd had congestion issues since I was a child, and I really hadn't thought much could be done about it, but if something could have been done, I would have welcomed the change. I also developed a very bad case of acid reflux. It had gotten so bad I could taste the acid in my throat all day long, and the discomfort would wake me from my sleep at night.

Through it all, my main concern was my lack of energy. It was just awful. I would wake up tired and stay tired throughout the day. I would fight my way through the tiredness, but it was always there.

I decided to remove poultry from my diet; as a result, I lost around twenty pounds, and my weight hovered around 180 pounds. I also gained some much-needed energy.

So the removal of pork, beef, and poultry from my diet made me a pescatarian. Though I did gain some energy as a result of my change in diet, I still woke up tired and fought tiredness throughout the day, though it wasn't as bad as it had been before. My acid reflux wasn't as bad either, but it was still an issue. I was still stricken with congestion issues, and I continually fought the flu and colds. Since I was doing better than before, I just chalked my remaining ailments up to getting older. I really didn't think it could get much better, and relatively speaking, I felt pretty good.

CHAPTER 13:

DECONSTRUCTING THE PLANT-BASED DIET

Though I was at a point where I was comfortable with my pescatarian diet and didn't think there was much more that I could do, I was still on the lookout for new knowledge that could improve my health. Shortly before I adopted a plant-based diet, I felt an urgency to find something that would once and for all deal with my congestion issues.

I decided to give a plant-based diet a try, and it was based on certain principles. I studied Dr. Sebi's methodology and researched why some people had successful outcomes and some people didn't when adopting a plant-based diet.

I reviewed different approaches toward eating the best plant-based foods, and I carefully studied the strengths and weaknesses of a plant-based diet. The result is I haven't been sick in four years since I adopted a plant-based diet. I haven't had a headache, toothache, cold, the flu, or pneumonia. I lost unhealthy weight, and my blood-pressure and cholesterol levels are excellent. I have just been healthy and full of energy. There are many vegans who enjoy these same benefits, and there are some who don't, because of how they approach the diet and way of life.

HYBRIDIZATION AND GENETIC MANIPULATION

Based on Dr. Sebi's methodology, I avoided eating hybrid-plant foods, even though they were plant foods. I followed Dr. Sebi's nutritional guide that excluded hybrid and GMO foods, in conjunction with taking African biomineral herbs to restore homeostasis in my body.[97] Hybridization is a process where two or more plants combine to form a new plant. Sometimes this is a natural process. Some of the original natural composition of nutrients is lost during this process, though. Most hybridization is a manufactured process that involves grafting plants that wouldn't occur naturally. Some of these hybridizations and genetic manipulations form mutations that are harmful.

Common-hybrid and GMO plant foods such as common wheat were left off the guide because they are harmful. Many people today have wheat- and gluten-related illnesses, and the number keeps growing. People have consumed wheat for thousands of years, but it is not until present times that wheat consumption has become problematic. The likely culprit is the hybridization and genetic modification of wheat that has produced common wheat.

Common wheat's hybridization and genetic modification turned wheat from an alkaline-forming food into an acid-forming food. Its genetic composition has also changed from being in line with supporting homeostasis to harming homeostasis. Common wheat had been hybridized to produce more gluten and to alter its gluten composition, which is likely a reason for the rise of wheat and gluten illnesses. Most common wheat has short stems, which is the result of RHt-dwarfing genes being introduced into wheat.[98, 99] Norman Borlaug inserted RHt genes into modern wheat varieties in the 1960s. These modifications to wheat's genetic structure make it different from the wheat people subsisted on for thousands of years and are the likely reasons for its negative impact on people's health. Avoidance of hybrid foods and sticking to consumption of foods on the nutritional guide is a major differentiator in the way I approach a plant-based diet compared to some other people's approach.

PROCESSED FOODS

The type of veganism that people practice also impacts their health benefits. There are two types of vegans—ethical vegans and dietary vegans. Ethical vegans don't eat animal products because they feel it is animal cruelty. Dietary vegans don't eat animal products because animal products are detrimental to good health. Dietary vegans are more concerned with eating the best plant-based foods that will support health, but ethical vegans might not be concerned with eating the healthiest foods. The latter may eat a lot of processed and junk plant-based food, and this can be as harmful as a diet heavily centered on meat.

Processed plant-based foods can contain one or more harmful additives than can include partially hydrogenated oils, processed carbohydrates, high-fructose corn syrup, synthetic sugars, additives, or preservatives. Types of processed foods—including meat—are hamburgers, hotdogs, candy, pastries, fast food, processed-grain cereals, and energy drinks.[100] The processing of plant-based foods either alters the plant product's life-sustaining components, or adds foreign substances that cause harm to the body.

PARTIALLY HYDROGENATED OILS

Natural vegetable oils are processed and manipulated to produce artificial trans fats called partially hydrogenated oils. Hydrogen is added to vegetable oils to make them more solid, give them a more desirable taste and texture, make them more tolerable to deep-frying, and add shelf life to foods. Partially hydrogenated oils are the primary source of trans fats in the Standard American Diet (SAD), even with the FDA instituting trans-fat food labeling in late 2006.[101] The FDA's initiative has helped reduce the consumption of trans fat, but many people do still heavily consume this health-harming substance.

The consumption of partially hydrogenated oils raises low-density lipoprotein (LDL) cholesterol and lowers high-density lipoprotein

(HDL) cholesterol.[102, 103, 104, 105] Consuming partially hydrogenated oils increase the risk of developing heart disease and stroke.[106] Heart disease is the number-one killer in the United States, accounting for 25 percent of all deaths.[107] LDL cholesterol in itself is not the cause of heart disease, and LDL is actually needed to support cell function. LDL cholesterol has been termed "bad" cholesterol because it becomes a problem when there is too much of it in the body. HDL cholesterol is low in fat and high in protein and acts as a vacuum, picking up excess LDL cholesterol as it travels through the bloodstream.

The body makes all the cholesterol it needs, and the consumption of cholesterol is not necessary and has detrimental consequences. The SAD diet is high in cholesterol and fat, and some of the consumed HDL cholesterol gets stuck on artery walls and threatens their integrity and homeostasis. This triggers the body's immune system to send out white blood cells to remove the LDL cholesterol sticking to artery walls. White blood cells envelop the LDL cholesterol in order to neutralize and remove it from artery walls and in the process convert it into a toxic, oxidized form of cholesterol.

Over time, more LDL cholesterol, white blood cells, and other cells stick to the compromised area of the artery walls and start a process of chronic inflammation that further harms the artery wall. The combination of these cells and compounds form a plaque on the artery wall that builds over time, stiffens and weakens the artery wall, and blocks the transportation of blood through the artery.[108] This inhibits the transportation of oxygen and nutrients, starving organs of energy and nutrients to support metabolic processes. Partially hydrogenated oil not only increases LDL cholesterol but also makes it smaller and denser and even more detrimental to sustaining homeostasis.

The consumption of partially hydrogenated oil poses a strong health risk, and in response, the FDA stepped in and made its inclusion on food labels mandatory to make the public aware of the potential health risk of the foods they were purchasing. Who allowed harmful substances like partially hydrogenated oils to make their way in food in the first place? You may be surprised to know that it is left up to the manufacturers of these substances to determine if they are safe.

"GENERALLY RECOGNIZED AS SAFE" (GRAS) FOOD ADDITIVES ARE NOT NECESSARILY SAFE

Along with the FDA making the food labeling of partially hydrogenated oil mandatory in 2006, in 2013 the US Food and Drug Administration went a step further and set in motion its plan to eliminate trans fats from processed foods. The FDA cited a CDC statistic that the elimination of partially hydrogenated oils from the food supply "could prevent 10,000–20,000 heart attacks and 3,000–7,000 coronary heart disease deaths each year in the United States.[109] As part of the 2013 initiative, the FDA removed partially hydrogenated oil's "Generally Recognized as Safe (GRAS)" status.[110] Partially hydrogenated oil was given the GRAS status that allowed it to be added to processed food. An important question that should be asked is, "How did this harmful substance get this status in the first place?"

Most of the public accepts that the food additives they eat are healthy, since they are allowed in food. Most would think there are checks and balances in place to stop harmful substances from being added to food. This is not the case though. Manufacturers of food additives determine if their additives are GRAS and are safe for consumption. There are no checks and balances in place to verify that the additives are actually safe. Food-additive manufacturers also do not have to inform the FDA or the public that they had developed a food additive and that only they determined it to be safe.[111, 112] This is a very dangerous process since a manufacturer would have no incentive to deny giving its own product the GRAS status, which would stop it from bringing its own product to market. This is not an isolated incident, and there are many other food additives, like the carbohydrate high-fructose corn syrup, that have been found to be harmful.[113]

THE LOW-CARB DIET, NATURAL CARBOHYDRATES, AND PROCESSED CARBOHYDRATES

There is a lot of confusion about whether carbohydrates in general are good or bad, and this is because of their association with processed carbohydrates. The low-carb diet was primarily responsible for putting all carbohydrates in the same "bad" basket. The association has undermined the benefits of a plant-based diet, because it is a high-carbohydrate diet. Low-carb diets became popular because they effectively supported short-term weight loss by avoiding carbohydrates in favor of animal-based protein and fat. Carbohydrate consumption became more associated with weight gain and obesity than did protein and even fat consumption.

Low-carb diets rightfully targeted the removal of processed and refined carbohydrates from the diet, because their consumption did have negative health consequences. But as word traveled through the grapevine about the strength of the low-carb diet, processed carbohydrates and refined carbohydrates simply became referred to as just "carbohydrates." The consumption of all carbohydrates became synonymous with weight gain.

Also, the detrimental properties of high-fructose corn syrup unfortunately became synonymous with all fructose, including the fructose in fruit. This was troubling because carbohydrates were the body's main fuel source, and fruit fructose made up a large percentage of that fuel. Many people have avoided eating fruits because they contain fructose due to fructose's association with high-fructose corn syrup and other additive sugars. Fruits, and the fructose they contain, are a natural food source that helps support homeostasis.

Fructose in Fruits

If you looked at the natural development of humankind and food gathering, fruits would have been the easiest food to gather. Fruits didn't need to be prepared, and you could walk up to a tree, pick a piece of fruit, and start eating. Raw, green vegetation was as easy to gather for consumption, but cooking it would have been more time consuming. Root vegetables and legumes would have been easy to secure also but would have taken the most time to prepare for consumption. Acquiring meat for consumption would have taken the most time and would have presented the most danger. From an acquisition standpoint, fruits would have logically been the bulk of the food consumed. Fruits also happened to be loaded with natural fructose that was digested quickly to support the body with quickly accessed energy for its fight-or-flight response in natural environments.

Fruits were also loaded with phytonutrients and antioxidants that combated disease and oxidative stress. Free radicals are atoms or groups of atoms that have an odd number of electrons. These atoms seek out cells to steal an electron to pair with their lone electrons. This causes oxidative stress, and it damages and ages the cells that the free radicals come in contact with. Antioxidants in fruits provide the extra electrons that the free radicals seek, saving healthy cells from being damaged.

Fruits also provided needed fiber that helped support the digestive tract and the digestion of food. Fiber bulked up stool so the muscles of the intestines did not have to strain to move the stool through the intestines. Continuous muscle strain in the intestines could rupture the mucous membrane that lined the intestine. These ruptures, called diverticula, collect waste that becomes putrefied over time.[114] The putrefied waste attacks the tissues of the intestines and releases toxins into the bloodstream.

Fiber not only protects the digestive tract but also aids in digestion and in supporting the immune system. Helpful bacteria in the digestive tract feeds on insoluble fiber and produces beneficial short-chain fatty acids that have numerous beneficial properties that include lowering the pH level in the colon and increasing the absorption of minerals.[115] Helpful bacteria also unbind polyphenols that are stuck to the insoluble fiber, allowing their absorption into the bloodstream. Polyphenols are phytonutrients, and numerous studies have shown that phytonutrients support the immune system.[116, 117, 118]

High-Fructose Corn Syrup

Fructose in fruits was naturally packaged by God/The Source/Nature to support a variety of functions in the body. The fiber, sugar, phytonutrients, and other compounds worked together in a way that created synergy and was supportive of connected functions. High-fructose corn syrup (HFCS) was made just to be an energy source. Since HFCS was not packaged with components that controlled its absorption into the bloodstream, HFCS entered the bloodstream and abnormally spiked the blood-sugar level.

HFCS is in most processed foods that use sweeteners, since it is sweeter and is cheaper to produce. HFCS could be found in soda, candy, cookies, cakes, hot dogs, pastries, ice cream, yogurt, bread, salad dressings, canned fruit, cereal bars, cereal, boxed processed macaroni, energy drinks, and more.

High consumption of HFCS had been linked to weight gain, type 2 diabetes, metabolic syndrome, and high triglyceride levels, all of which increase the risk of heart disease. The article "Metabolic Dangers of High-Fructose Corn Syrup"[119] addressed the detrimental effects of HFCS consumption, and the article also served to highlight the issue of confusion that arises when speaking or writing about HFCS and fructose.

The article was clearly about the dangers of HFCS, but the article also referred to it as "dietary fructose" or simply "fructose." Reading "dietary fructose" and "fructose" out of context, one could have easily associated the findings with all fructose. I encountered this issue with many articles I have read on high-fructose corn syrup and conversations I have had on the subject.

Not only was the consumption HFCS problematic because it was used as an additive sugar, its chemical makeup was also problematic. Mercury-cell technology was used in the production of HFCS, which leached toxic mercury into the HFCS.[120] The Corn Refiners Association tried to assure the public that mercury-free processing had replaced the mercury technology. Despite the Corn Refiners

Association's assurances, further research showed that mercury-cell technology was still in use in certain factories.

There had been a big downslide of consumer confidence regarding HFCS because of studies that showed the harmful effects of HFCS consumption. Industry addressed the issue by modifying its HFCS product and renaming it, which disassociated it with HFCS. The newer HFCS-90 contained 90 percent processed fructose instead of the 42 or 55 percent fructose of HFCS, which allowed it to be simply named "fructose" or "fructose syrup."[121]

This manipulation added to the confusion as to what was and was not fructose, and all fructose became bad in the minds of many people. This was very disturbing because fruit consumption is vitally important in supporting homeostasis in the body, and many people chose to forgo its consumption, thinking its fructose was harmful.

Refined Complex Carbs

Refined complex carbohydrates also gave carbohydrates a bad name. Complex carbs are starches and fiber, and refined complex carbs are the starches with the fiber removed. The refining process not only removed fiber but also removed much of the food's nutritional value, including vitamins, minerals, phytonutrients, and healthy oils. Breads, pasta, cereal, candy, pastries, cakes, cookies, and pies made from enriched and bleach flours are all examples of refined complex carbs.[122]

Refined complex carbs often contained refined sugars, including HFCS, and processed fat, including partially hydrogenated oil. The heavy consumption of refined complex carbs also led to weight gain, type 2 diabetes, metabolic syndrome, and high triglyceride levels, all of which increased the risk of heart disease.

Complex Carbs and Simple Carbs

The consumption of natural complex carbs and simple carbs can be supportive of health. Practitioners of a plant-based diet have consumed these carbs in different amounts, depending on their philosophical approach. Natural simple carbs, fruits, were digested quickly, which minimized the amount of time they remained in the body. This helped greatly to regulate weight gain and kept energy levels constantly high. Consumption of large amounts of simple carbs supported the philosophy of eating five to six small meals a day to promote high energy and metabolism and to reduce strain put on the digestive system.

Natural complex carbs, grains and legumes, were digested more slowly, and since they stayed in the body longer, they had more of a chance to go through the whole glucose-conversion process and contribute to weight gain.[123] Both simple carbs and complex were converted to glucose for energy and were stored as glycogen in the liver and muscles. After glycogen storage became full in the muscles and liver, excess complex carbs were converted to triglycerides and were stored in fats cells.[124]

All starchy foods were not created equal. The consumption of foods like quinoa and garbanzo beans that was high in resistant starch (RS) was preferable to starchy foods like white potatoes because of their high glycemic load.[125] The resistant starch in quinoa was digested in the colon by intestinal bacteria, instead of in the small intestine like the starch that is converted into glucose in white potatoes. The beneficial bacteria's digestion of resistant starch produced short-chain fatty acids such acetate, butyrate, and propionate feed the cells of the colon and other organs. The production of short-chain fatty acids in the colon[126, 127] resulted in stimulating blood flow to the colon, absorption of minerals into the bloodstream, and the inhibition of the growth of harmful bacteria. A diet of natural complex and simple carbs that promotes high energy, easy digestion, a strong digestive tract, and weight loss and control would consist of mostly simple carbs attained from eating whole fruit, and a small quantity of complex carbs from foods like quinoa and garbanzo beans that contain more resistant starch.

VEGETABLES AND MICRONUTRIENTS

Simple and complex carbs are the body's main sources of energy, called macronutrients. Fruits and root vegetables are concentrated with carbohydrate energy macronutrients and contain micronutrients to a lesser degree. Green leafy vegetables contain carbohydrate energy macronutrients to a lesser degree, and vitamins, minerals, and phytonutrients to a larger degree. Vegetables are the primary source of micronutrients in a whole-food, plant-based diet. Vegetables in a well-balanced whole-food, plant-based diet deliver all the vitamins and minerals that are needed to support homeostasis, and there is no need to supplement with vitamins, except vitamin B12. Vegans, vegetarians, and carnivores all likely can benefit from vitamin B12 supplementation.

Vegetables, like amaranth, kale, mustard greens, onions, and sea vegetables, are the most concentrated micronutrient plant-based foods. Vegetables are best sources for micronutrients and are specifically better sources for micronutrients than vitamin supplementation. The natural combinations of nutrients put in place by God/The Source/Nature in vegetables produce synergy that doses of single nutrients do not provide. Science in fact shows that unnatural concentrations of nutrients can lead to higher rates of mortality, and supplementing with single synthetic nutrient vitamin A, vitamin B, and beta-carotene all increased mortality compared to no supplementation.[128, 129, 130]

Vitamin B12 Supplementation May Be Necessary for Many

The proper level of vitamin B12 is vital for supporting homeostasis in the body. Vitamin B12 is needed to break down carbohydrates and fats and supports the replication of DNA to generate new healthy cells. Vitamin B12, iron, and folate are used together to produce hemoglobin and new red blood cells. Vitamin B12 plays an essential role is chemical reactions that maintain the myelin coating that protects the spinal, cranial and peripheral nerves.

Vitamin B12 used to be readily available in nature, and there was no need to think about supplementation. Synthetic processes have all but eliminated the natural sources of vitamin B12 in the soil and water sources that God/The Source/Nature provided to help maintain homeostasis in living beings. Beneficial microbes in soil manufacture vitamin B12 from the element cobalt in soil. These microbes were bountiful in the soil and were washed off the land into water sources like rivers, streams, and lakes. Current industrial farming, food production, and water-purification methods destroy the beneficial microbes and the vitamin B12 they produce.

Farming methods use antimicrobial chemicals to kill pathogens on crops, which also kill the beneficial bacteria that produce vitamin B12. This results in the reduction of beneficial microbes and their vitamin B12 that is attached to crops, and it also reduces the amount found in the soil. The reduction of microbes in the soil means the reduction of microbes washed off the land into water sources. Food-production methods used to kill pathogens and to sanitize food crops on the production line also kill the beneficial bacteria.[131] The public is also cautioned to thoroughly wash produce before consuming them to remove residual chemicals that remain on the produce. This also washes off vitamin B12. Public water is treated with chemicals to kill pathogens, and unfortunately, they also kill the beneficial vitamin B12–producing bacteria.

Meat, fortified foods, and supplements have become the reliable sources of vitamin B12. Even with meat consumption being available to carnivores, and fortified foods being available to a wide portion of the US population, up to 15 percent of the population has vitamin B12–deficiency.[132] If you take into consideration the people who are not deficient but are just low in vitamin B12, the number becomes even more troublesome.

Vitamin B12–supplementation becomes a tricky subject and not because of the reduction of vitamin B12–sources. Under normal circumstances, the body needs relatively small amounts of vitamin B12, and the body does a very good job recycling its own stores of vitamin

B12. "Vitamin B12 is excreted in the bile and is effectively reabsorbed. This is known as enterohepatic circulation. The amount of B12 excreted in the bile can vary from 1 to 10ug (micrograms) a day. People on diets low in B12, including vegans and some vegetarians, may be obtaining more B12 from reabsorption than from dietary sources. Reabsorption is the reason it can take over twenty years for a deficiency disease to develop."[133]

The diminishing of vitamin B12 food sources may not be the major reason or reason at all for vitamin B12–deficiency. The issue may be solely an absorption issue that may make supplementation necessary to counteract the absorption issue.[134] Autoimmune atrophic gastritis (AG) is an autoimmune disease where antibodies attack stomach cells that produce the mucoprotein called intrinsic factor. Intrinsic factor must combine with vitamin B12 in order for the body to absorb vitamin B12. If the production of intrinsic factor is reduced or nonexistent, then vitamin B12 will be minimally absorbed by the body or not absorbed at all.

This can lead to the development of megaloblastic anemia, neurological disorders, and nerve damage. Antibiotics—either taking them or consuming meat and milk that contain them—heavy alcohol consumption, prolonged antacid use, smoking, and prolonged and extreme stress also cause or support the development of vitamin B12 deficiency.[135, 136]

There is still plenty of debate left about whether a person who is healthy and has a healthy digestive tract needs to worry about consuming enough vitamin B12. There is some evidence that supports the idea that the body can produce vitamin B12 in the small intestine.[137] This, combined with the body's ability to recycle vitamin B12 from the colon, would minimize concerns about the reduction of vitamin B12 in the food supply. The issue may solely be with people who have autoimmune diseases that affect the absorption of vitamin B12 and people who consume drugs and toxins that affect vitamin B12 absorption. The logical route for healthy people who don't want to supplement with vitamin B12 to determine if supplementation is necessary would be to take periodic blood tests to monitor their vitamin B12–levels without supplementation. If the B12 store isn't diminished without supplementation, then supplementation isn't needed. If the B12 store diminished quickly, then B12 supplementation is needed.

VITAMIN D AND HEALTH

God/The Source/Nature designed people to have a very nurturing and healing relationship with the sun. In the relationship with the sun, exposure to sunlight provides people with vitamin D.

The body converts cholesterol in the body to vitamin D when the skin is exposed to sunlight's UVB radiation. The body also makes all the cholesterol it needs from fat, so neither vitamin D nor cholesterol acquisition is left up to food consumption. The sun is our natural source of vitamin D, not plant or animal food. Vitamin D's role in the body is so important that God/The Source/Nature did not leave vitamin D acquisition solely dependent on food consumption. Vitamin D is involved in so many of the body's functions that it may be the most important vitamin for supporting overall health.

Vitamin D regulates hundreds of genes in the human body, by binding to the vitamin D receptors in cells. These receptors are found in cells all throughout the body, including breasts, bones, brain, heart, immune system, intestines, kidneys, ovaries, prostate, parathyroid gland, skin, and testicles.[138] Vitamin D supports bone growth and healing by regulating calcium and phosphorous levels in the blood.

Vitamin D regulates the immune system and turns down the immune response to combat autoimmune diseases like lupus, multiple sclerosis, and rheumatoid arthritis. Vitamin D also activates the immune system to fight cancer, influenza, pneumonia, and tuberculosis, and pneumonia. Vitamin D also fights diabetes by modifying insulin response and release and also decreases cardiovascular risks such as heart attacks and strokes.[139, 140, 141]

Many people are cautious about getting their needed vitamin D from the sun, and with good reason. The pollution that industry has created has thrown off the natural balance of compounds and elements in the atmosphere that God/The Source/Nature had established. The balance of compounds and elements in the ozone layer protected the earth and people from excessive exposure to the sun's radiation. Pollutants like chlorofluorocarbons have depleted and have produced holes in the ozone layer, letting excessive radiation now reach the earth. The increase in radiation has led to the increased risk of developing skin cancer, so people are cautioned not to stay in the sun for long periods and to use sunblock to reduce the absorption of UVB radiation. Organizations have developed recommendations for how long to stay in the sun, but these recommendations are problematic because they are developed from studying the reaction of pale skin to UVB radiation. Darker skin can withstand higher and longer periods of sun exposure, and need longer exposure than pale skin to produce the needed levels of vitamin D.

Getting Vitamin D from the Sun

The body is capable of making up to 10,000 IUs of vitamin D from sun exposure, and after maximum UVB exposure, the vitamin D precursors in the skin reach a tipping point and any additional vitamin D from the sun is not used.[142] Ten thousand IUs of vitamin D is equal to 250 mcg, 100 ng/ml, and 250 nmol/L of vitamin D. The ng/ml and nmol/L are units used for testing blood vitamin D levels. The body will stop using the vitamin D it makes after 10,000 IUs or 100 ng/ml.

In spite of the natural daily limit of vitamin D production established by God/The Source/Nature, organizations have developed their own recommendations for vitamin D levels. The Vitamin D Council lists 40–80 ng/ml as sufficient, 31–39 ng/ml as insufficient, and 0–30 ng/ml as deficient vitamin D levels.[143] The Endocrine Society lists 30–100 ng/ml as sufficient, 21–29 ng/ml as insufficient, and 0–20 as deficient.[144] The Food and Nutrition Board lists 20 ng/ml and higher as sufficient, 12–20 ng/ml as insufficient, and 0–11 ng/ml as deficient.[145] Testing laboratories list 32–100 ng/ml as sufficient and 0–31 ng/ml as deficient. I work to keep my vitamin D level between 75–100 ng/ml, and closer to 100 ng/ml.

UV Index, Skin Type, and Vitamin D Production

UV stands for ultraviolet, and the UV Index is the international standard measurement of the strength of the sun's ultraviolet radiation reaching the earth. The UV Index will be different depending on your location and the particular time of the day. The UV Index rises through the day and decreases through the afternoon. The UV Index is strongest between 10:00 a.m. and 2:00 p.m. The UV Index was developed to protect people against excessive ultraviolet-light exposure that can result in sunburns, eye damage, skin aging, and skin cancer.

The UV Index is a scale from zero to eleven in relation to the strength of the sun's UV rays reaching the earth, and it contains five category recommendations. It is important to keep in mind the recommendations were given for adults with pale to lightly tan skin that contains lower levels of UV-protecting melanin. Children with pale to lightly tan skin who are sensitive to the sun need to take extra precautions.

UV Index Recommendations

Recommendations are based on fair to lightly tanned skin.[146]

UV Index	Description	Recommended Protection
0–2	Low danger from the sun's UV rays for the average person	Wear sunglasses on bright days, use broad-spectrum SPF 30+ sunscreen on sensitive skin
3–5	Moderate risk of harm from	Stay in shade near midday

	unprotected sun exposure	when the sun is strongest, wear protective clothing if you are outside, wear spectrum SPF 30+ sunscreen
6–7	High risk of harm from unprotected sun exposure	Reduce time in the sun between 10:00 a.m. and 4:00 p.m., wear protective clothing if you are outside, wear spectrum SPF 30+ sunscreen
8–10	Very high risk of harm from unprotected sun exposure	Minimize time in the sun between 10:00 a.m. and 4:00 p.m., wear protective clothing if you are outside, wear spectrum SPF 30+ sunscreen
11+	Extreme risk of harm from unprotected sun exposure	Avoid sun exposure between two hours before and after noon, wear protective clothing outside, a wide-brimmed hat, and UV-blocking sunglasses.

Skin Type and Sun Exposure

Darker-skinned people traditionally inhabited warmer climates, and the larger melanin content in their skin allowed them to spend more time in the sun without suffering adverse effects. The extra protection of their melanin strongly managed UV absorption, which caused vitamin D production to occur over a longer period.

Lighter-skinned people traditionally inhabited colder climates with a lower UVI and wore more clothing, so their skin was less exposed to the sun. The lack of melanin allowed for the quicker absorption of UV radiation and the faster production of vitamin D. The differences in skin type dictate the different amounts of UV protection the skin offers and the amount sun exposure needed for maximum levels of vitamin D production.

Chart based on Dermato Endocrinology's study.[147]

Skin Type	UVI 0–2	UVI 3–5	UVI 6–7	UVI 8–10 Tanning	UVI 11+
Lightest— Never Tan	None	10–15 minutes	5–10 minutes	2–8 minutes	1–5 minutes
Rarely Tan	None	15–20 minutes	10–15 minutes	5–8 minutes	2–8 minutes
Slowly Tan	None	20–30 minutes	15–20 minutes	10–15 minutes	5–10 minutes
Rapidly Tan	None	30–40 minutes	20–30 minutes	15–20 minutes	10–15 minutes
Darkest— Always Dark	None	40–60 minutes	30–40 minutes	20–30 minutes	15–20 minutes

Vitamin D2 or Vitamin D3

It best to get vitamin D from sun exposure. Many people spend most of their days working in buildings and are not able to get out in the sun to make the needed amount of vitamin D. Is it very important to get the required amounts of vitamin D, so as a last resort occasional supplementation may be necessary?

Vitamin D supplements come in two forms, vitamin D3 and vitamin D2. Most D3 supplements are animal-based and D2 supplements are plant-based. D2 had been used for years without any issue, but recommended usage has switched to D3. Studies show that the skin produces D3, which has now positioned D3 as being the better supplement. This put vegans and vegetarians who felt it necessary to supplement in the compromising position of taking the animal-based D3 over the plant-based D2. Fortunately, a non-animal-based form of D3 was found recently. It was discovered that the lichen microorganism produces D3, so now a vegan vitamin D3 is now also available. Unfortunately, the vegan D3 is not as available for purchase as is the D2 version.

The D2 version shouldn't be thrown out the window, because it is still effective but just not as effective as D3. The liver converts both D2 and D3 into calcidiol, also known as 25-hydroxycholecalciferol, or 25-hydroxyvitamin D, and is abbreviated 25(OH)D. The body converts D3 into 25(OH)D more efficiently, so a larger amount D2 is needed to raise 25(OH)D to the same level. D3 also has a longer half-life in the body and longer shelf life in supplements compared to D2. Putting this issue in perspective, D2 supplementation is still a viable option. More D2 is needed to raise 25(OH)D levels, but with concentration of D2 in supplements, this is not a big issue. Shelf life is not a big issue if you are spreading usage of years.

VEGETABLE FAT AND VEGETABLE PROTEIN

Fat and protein consumption is essential for supporting metabolic processes and homeostasis. The God/The Source/Nature designed patterns in the body that only require 10 percent of the diet to be from fat and protein. A well-balanced whole-food, plant-based diet provides this ratio. Fat is needed to protect brain and nerve health, transport fat-soluble vitamins, and to form hormones. Protein is needed for antibody and enzyme production, to build cells, transport molecules, and transmit messages throughout the body.[148]

Though fat and protein performs vital functions, they are needed at a far smaller percentage than carbohydrates. Science has shown that excessive fat consumption leads to various health problems that include stroke, high blood pressure, heart disease, cancer, and osteoporosis. Excessive animal-based protein consumption has also been linked to increased rates of cancer and illness.

GENETICALLY MODIFIED ORGANISMS' (GMO) EFFECTS ON OUR HEALTH

GMOs are genetically modified organisms and are the direct manipulation of genes in foods. Eighty percent of genetic modification to crops is done to make them resistant to pesticides. A smaller percentage of genetic manipulation is done to make the look and smell of products more appealing to consumers. GMOs exist outside the natural law of God/The Source/Nature. They did not develop in response to the natural order and energy of life. Their composition is not seen as natural to the body.

The argument of the bioengineers is the genetic manipulation only affects the targeted trait of the food and nothing else. The reality is bioengineers don't know that is true, because they don't know how the change affects every other trait and component of the manipulated food. Components in the food we eat develop in relation to each other, and bioengineers have no idea how manipulating one gene affects others and how the consumption of the modified food affects the body. GMO foods often make their way to the food supply without the proper third-party long-term studies being performed to determine the health consequences of genetic modification.

Gilles-Eric Seralini[149] performed a study of the long-term effects of Monsanto's GMO corn, which was already approved and in the market place. He fed rats Monsanto's Roundup Ready corn, and they developed very large tumors, and some died. The study was published in the journal *Food and Chemical Toxicology*. Seralini faced an onslaught of criticism because he supposedly used rats that had a tendency to develop tumors (the Sprague-Dawley strain), and he used too few rats. The journal retracted the study, and the scientific community sanctioned the industry-driven censorship.[150]

Interestingly enough Seralini performed the same study Monsanto used to get the GMO corn approved. Seralini used the same strain of rats and the same number of rats as the Monsanto study did. The Seralini study was also published in the same journal as the Monsanto study. The difference being Seralini ran his study for a longer period. Monsanto's short-term study showed no evidence of abnormal tumor development, while Seralini's long-term study gave showed that the Monsanto study was stopped prematurely and didn't give enough time for the tumors to develop.

Through maneuverings like getting the Seralini study retracted, the debate as to whether GMOs are harmful continues. Some would argue that the genetic manipulation might not be harmful, but it is apparent that the GMO crops engineered to be resistant to pesticides are harmful and that involves 80 percent of GMO foods. Crops like soy are GMO engineered to be resistant to toxic pesticides, which allows them to be sprayed directly with the toxic pesticides. These crops end up in the marketplace, contaminated with large amounts of harmful pesticide residue.[151, 152]

Clinical tests have shown that Monsanto's Ready Roundup pesticide has harmful toxic and hormonal effects.[153] Previous tests done on animals had shown that glyphosate, the main ingredient in Roundup, negatively affected embryonic development, disrupted hormones, and interfered with male fertility. More recent tests were done using the isolated glyphosate, and those tests showed that glyphosate by itself didn't have much of a toxic effect on human cells. Though glyphosate is the main ingredient in Roundup, it is not the only ingredient. The other ingredients in Roundup allow the glyphosate to penetrate human cells and cause damage.[154] Roundup was found to be 125 times more toxic than its active ingredient glyphosate and was among the most toxic pesticide products tested, though it is commonly believed that Roundup is among the safest herbicides used.[155]

The legal level for residue levels of glyphosate in foods had been at 0.1 to 0.2 milligrams per kilogram. The residue levels of glyphosate found in GMO soy crops exceed the legal limits by an average of 2,000 percent.[156] Though the argument continues as to whether modifying the genetic structure of food is dangerous to the body, it is evident that pesticide-resistant GMO crops are harmful.

CHAPTER 14:

THE CHINA PROJECT—DISEASES OF AFFLUENCE AND DIETARY LIFESTYLE

In 1970, Chinese premier Zhou Enlai was diagnosed with cancer, and he commissioned a cross-sectional account of death rates by disease and counties across China. This collection of data was called the Cancer Atlas and consisted of data on 880 million people, which was about 95 percent of the population. The data showed that cancer was localized to different areas of China, which suggested that cancer was caused by dietary and environmental factors and was not caused by any genetics.

The Cancer Atlas presented Dr. Campbell and his colleagues with compelling information and the chance to investigate the relationship between cancer and diet in human beings. In 1980, Dr. Campbell and his colleagues began their famous epidemiological study called "The China Project." Dr. Campbell along with his colleagues from Cornell University, Oxford University, and the Chinese government devised the study to analyze patterns of disease across China and dietary and lifestyle factors that influenced the diseases.

Dr. Campbell and his team's study included 6,500 Chinese adults across sixty-five counties in China. Participants had to answer dietary and lifestyle questions and supply blood and urine to be tested for nutrient concentrations, diseases, and toxins. The researchers also collected food samples, analyzed geographical factors, and collected data that resulted in 367 variables being analyzed as part of the study. Dr. Campbell and his team found there was a correlation between types of diseases and wealth.

Chronic and degenerative diseases tended to occur in affluent areas and were labeled "diseases of affluence." The diseases were attributed to "nutritional extravagance" that involved the excessive consumption of processed foods and meat. Diseases of affluence consisted of chronic, non-communicable diseases, such as cancer, asthma, obesity, cardiovascular disease, type 2 diabetes, high blood pressure, osteoporosis, colorectal cancer, acne, depression, hypertension, diseases related to vitamin and mineral deficiencies, gout, and some type of allergies.

There was also a correlation between poverty and disease. "Diseases of poverty" were due to nutritional inadequacy and poor sanitation. These diseases include malnutrition, communicable disease like tuberculosis, AIDS/HIV, and parasitic diseases like malaria. Contaminated water, inadequate sanitation, and poor health care were factors that related to the spread of diseases among poorer populations.

Chinese people who lived in rural areas who ate whole-food, plant-based diets or ate close to it, in general, didn't suffer from diseases of affluence or diseases of poverty. Dr. Campbell and his team also found that Chinese women who ate a plant-based diet had lower levels of estrogen, and lower levels of estrogen were related to lower levels of breast cancer. Interestingly, lower levels of estrogen caused menses to happen later in life and menopause to happen earlier. This kept childbearing years to periods of higher mental and social stability, and physical vitality. The team also found a positive relationship between high fiber consumption and lower rates of colon and rectal cancer. The results were so consistent across demographics that Dr. Campbell and his team concluded the closer people came to eating a plant-based diet, the lower their risk for developing chronic disease and the higher the chance of supporting homeostasis.

The data made them realize that even small differences in the amounts of animal protein in people's diets raised the incidence of disease. "After data from the project was analyzed, he reached a new level of confidence in his conclusions, solidifying his theory that plant-based foods, as a class, promoted health, whereas animal-based foods, as a class, carried health risks."[157]

CHRONIC INFLAMMATION

Chronic inflammation is the linchpin of diseases of affluence. The continuous consumption of toxic substances triggers the health-supporting acute-inflammation process, but it doesn't allow it to turn off. Acute inflammation is the immune response that increases blood flow to capillaries in an area of the body that has been injured or infected. The process includes dilation and increased permeability of the blood vessels that allows increased blood flows to deliver more fluids, proteins, white blood cells (neutrophils, eosinophils, and or macrophages), and proinflammatory cells to the affected area. This action localizes the infected or injured tissue, causing inflammation or swelling in the area to maximize the healing process. Under normal circumstances, the acute inflammation is turned off after the infected or injured area has healed.

Chronic inflammation occurs when acute inflammation is not completely turned off because of the continuous onslaught of toxic material. Under this condition, proinflammatory cells are slowly and continuously released into the body and act like a slow-burning fire, slowly destroying the healthy cells they come in contact with. This continuous release of inflammatory cells supports the development of diseases of affluence. These toxic substances include environmental pollutants, recreational and pharmaceutical drugs, and excessive consumption of animal-based foods, processed foods, and chemically and genetically altered foods.

These foods do not present combinations of nutrients that develop in response to the natural patterns of energy established by

God/The Source/Nature. The substances are seen as foreign, not totally compatible with the body, or too much of a particular substance that throws of homeostasis.

THE SKINNY ABOUT FAT AND INFLAMMATION

Fat is good for you, and it is vital for healthy living, but too much fat is detrimental to homeostasis. Excess fat consumption leads to a host of diseases that include coronary heart disease, atherosclerosis, gallstones, high blood pressure, osteoarthritis, and type 2 diabetes. In the natural proportions that whole plant-based foods provide, fat plays key roles in supporting homeostasis.

Most know fat serves as a secondary energy source, but it also stores fat-soluble vitamins A, D, E, and K, and insulates the body. Fat works with proteins to transmit messages throughout the body. It is used to build cell membranes and regulate cell metabolism and division. Fat is also part of the immune system's inflammation process. The Western diet is loaded with fat, especially proinflammatory fat that supports chronic inflammation.

Omega-6 acid linoleic acid (LA) fatty acids are generally thought of as being proinflammatory, while omega-3 acid alpha-linoleic acid (ALA) fatty acids are thought of as being anti-inflammatory. To support homeostasis, there should be a balance of 2:1–4:1, omega-6 to omega-3,[158] but the Western diet consists of a ratio from 16:1 to 50:1. Dr. Campbell noted that indigenous cultures throughout the world that are free from processed foods have a ratio of 1:1. The Western diet is extremely proinflammatory because of the large consumption of meat and omega-6 dominant oils used in food preparation. For instance, safflower oil has a ratio of 75:0.1, sunflower oil 71:0.6, and corn oil 57:1.[159]

The high consumption of proinflammatory omega-6 fatty acids throws off the delicate balance and supports chronic inflammation. Trans fats are also proinflammatory and are used in a variety of processed foods that include cakes, cereals, cookies, crackers, fast food,

French fries, fried chicken, frozen-dinner food, ground beef, ice cream, margarine, muffins, pancakes, pies and pie crusts, shortening, and waffles.

Aside from the complementary proinflammatory and anti-inflammatory properties of omega-6 and omega-3 fatty acids, they are complementary in other aspects also. Omega-6 raises blood pressure, while omega-3 reduces blood pressure. Omega-6 oxidizes arterial cholesterol, while omega-3's antioxidant properties prevents oxidation. Omega-6 promotes blood clotting, while omega-3 work against blood clotting. Omega-6 and omega-3 fatty acids also produce complementary hormone messengers.[160] In nature, opposite forces work together in a complementary nature, and the relationship between omega-6 and omega-3 exemplifies this nature.

CHAPTER 15:

THE GOD-AWAKENING DIET (GAD)

I follow a highly alkaline, non-hybrid plant-based diet consisting of mostly whole plant foods. The nutritional guide listed is based on the non-hybrid plant foods recommended by the herbalist Dr. Sebi. Many commonly eaten foods are left off the list because they are hybrid, have a compromised or incomplete structure, and introduce compounds during digestion that harm the digestive tract. It is best to eat natural non-hybrid foods that have chemical affinity with the body, so when they are digested they don't produce harmful byproducts that compromise the immune system. 80% of the immune system is made up of helpful bacteria that live in the digestive tract, and foods that are completely recognized by the body support the healthy bacteria and immune system in the digestive tract.

NUTRITIONAL GUIDE

Items with an * are items I added that are not part of Dr. Sebi's regimen. I do find value in the items, though he excludes them.

Protein:

(*Almonds have recently been removed by Dr. Sebi after years of being on the list, because they were found to contain a

compound called amygdalin with contains bound and inert cyanide. The amygdalin compound has been found to target only cancer cells once in the bloodstream and is even considered to be a vitamin, vitamin B17. You can find information about amygdalin and the conspiracy surrounding it here: http://www.naturallifeenergy.com/conspiracy-behind-vitamin-b17-amygdalin-laetrile-cyanide-and-cancer-treatment/. I find value in almonds and have been to able to successfully reverse disease in my body while consuming almonds. Amygdalin is also found in many commonly eaten foods and herbs.)

Grains: Amaranth, Fonio, Kamut, Quinoa, Rye, Spelt, Tef, Wild Rice
Legumes: Garbanzo Beans (Chickpeas)
Nut & Seeds: *Almonds, Brazil Nuts, Hemp Seeds, Pine Nuts, Raw Sesame "Tahini" Butter, Walnuts

Milk:

Hemp seed milk, Coconut milk, Walnut milk, Almond milk (It is better to make your own milk than to buy it to make sure you are drinking pure nut or seed milk. See recipes.)

Energy

Fruits (Whole fruits and not canned fruits that are processed and contain cancer causing additives and preservatives)

Apples, Bananas, Berries, Cantaloupe, Cherries, Currants, Dates, Figs, Grapes -seeded, Key Limes, Mango, Melons -seeded, Oranges, Papayas, Peaches, Pears, Plums, Prickly Pear, Prunes, Raisins -seeded, Soft Jelly Coconuts, Soursops, Tamarind

Cleansing

Vegetables: Amaranth greens (Callaloo), Avocado, Bell Peppers, Chayote (Mexican Squash), Cucumber, Dandelion greens, Garbanzo beans (Chickpeas), Green Banana, Izote (cactus leaf), Kale, Lettuce (all, except Iceberg), Mushrooms (all, except Shitake), Mustard greens, Nopales, Okra, Olives, Onions Purslane (Verdolaga), Poke salad, Sea Vegetables (wakame/dulse/arame/hijiki/nori), Squash, Tomato (Cherry and Plum only), Tomatillo, Turnip greens, Watercress, Zucchini

Oils

(It is best to minimize the use of oils because they are not a whole foods and using too much oil can lead to inflammation, support the development of diabetes, and damage arteries)

Grape seed Oil (minimize use because it is high in omega-6), Sesame Oil, Hempseed Oil, Avocado Oil, Olive Oil (Better not to cook with – destroys integrity of the oil at high heat), Coconut Oil (Better not to cook with – destroys integrity of the oil at high heat)

Seasonings

Achiote, Basil, Bay leaf, Cayenne (African Bird Pepper), Cilantro, Coriander, Dill, Habanero, Marjoram, Onion Powder, Oregano, Parsley, Powdered Granulated Seaweed (Kelp/Dulce/Nori), Pure Sea Salt, Sage, Savory, Sweet Basil, Tarragon, Thyme

Herbal Teas

(It is better to drink herbal teas than regular tea, like green tea, because they don't contain caffeine and contain a wide range of phytonutrients that support the immune system)

Alvaca, Anise, Chamomile, Cloves, Fennel, Ginger, Lemon grass, Red Raspberry, Sea Moss Tea

Sugars

(As with oils you should minimize your consumption of additive sugar)

Date sugar is the best sugar to consume from a health point of view. Date sugar is simply dried and ground dates. All of its nutrients are intact (except for its water) which controls digestion of its sugar.

100% Pure Agave Syrup (from cactus) is good but its processing can compromise its carbohydrate structure

100% Pure Maple Syrup – Grade B recommended /Maple "Sugar" (from dried maple syrup) is good but harmful chemicals sometimes used to keep the whole in the tree open gets into the syrup

Along with following the nutritional guide, I also used herbs during the first three months of my conversion to a plant based diet.

Cleansing Herbs:

Items with an * are items I added that are not part of Dr. Sebi's regimen. I do find value in the items, though he excludes them. These are only a few of herbs Dr. Sebi uses to reverse disease, but these herbs are the foundational herbs in the process of healing. They clean and help restore the health of the liver and kidneys so they can clean the blood more effectively and reduce stress put on the organs. (These are also the safer combinations of herbs to use without having an in-depth understanding of herbalism.)

- Burdock root—blood and liver cleanser, diuretic[161]
- Bladderwrack (seaweed)—vitamin and mineral supplement
- *Black walnut—kills parasites
- *Black seed[162]
- *Bromelain and papain—dissolves proteins[163, 164]
- Chaparral leaf
- *Chlorella (algae)—protein, vitamin, and mineral supplement, detoxifier[165]
- *Curcumin—antioxidant, supports brain, cardiovascular, and joint health[166]
- Dandelion—blood and liver cleanser[167]

- Elderberry (*Sambucus nigra*)—strengthens the body against colds[168]
- Irish moss (seaweed)—vitamin and mineral supplement
- *Kalmegh leaf—*Andrographis paniculata*
- Kelp (seaweed)—vitamin and mineral supplement
- *Mullein—removes mucus in the small intestine[169]
- *Oil of oregano—antiviral
- Sage
- Sarsaparilla—blood purifier, diuretic, antibacterial, anti-inflammatory[170]
- *Wormwood leaf—kills parasites

HERBAL CLEANSE

During the first three months of my adoption of a plant-based diet I did an herbal cleanse. The main herbs I took on a daily basis were burdock root, dandelion, sarsaparilla, elderberry, bladderwrack, and Irish moss. These herbs target and clean the liver and kidneys, remove mucous from the body, and supply a wide variety of nutrients and phytonutrients that rejuvenate cells and stimulate the immune system. Halfway through the herbal cleanse, I added in bromelain and papain to dissolve protein stuck in the harmful mucus lining my small intestine, and mullein to remove built-up mucus. I did this so my body could more efficiently absorb nutrients through the intestinal wall into the bloodstream, so I would require less food to provide the nutrients my body needed. I also added black walnut and wormwood leaf to kill parasites in the colon.

SHORT-TERM JUMP-STARTER ORGAN CLEANSES

I also performed unconventional short-term organ cleanses for the liver-gallbladder and kidneys, to go along with a previously performed colon cleanse that I found to be very helpful. Many people face detox symptoms when converting to a plant-based diet, taking herbs, or a combination of them. A main reason for this is the colon is extremely unhealthy and cannot process waste correctly. This allows for toxins to back up and reenter the bloodstream, causing a spike in toxins that can lead to nausea and headaches.

It is very helpful to have a decently clean colon and kidneys before you start a general body detox. I was fortunate not to face any detox issues when I switched to a plant based diet, and did my herbal cleanse. Because of the number of people who have experienced detox symptoms who did not address cleaning their colons first, I attribute my colon cleanse with cleaning my colon enough so I didn't experience any significant backup of toxins. The colon cleanse I performed is a bit unconventional because unlike using plant foods and herbs only for the cleaning process, the cleanse used natural mineral deposits to pull putrid waste from the colon. Some people will shy away from ingesting this natural clay because it is not food and that is perfectly fine, but I felt the need to share my experience because it positively affected my health.

Colon Cleanse

The colon cleanse consisted of two main cleansing components, bentonite clay and psyllium husk. Bentonite clay[171, 172] is a volcanic ash that has been used to pull waste from pouches called diverticula that can develop in the intestinal walls.[173] These pouches form through the herniation of the mucous membrane lining the intestine wall, and the pouches collect waste that becomes putrid and difficult to remove. The putrid waste releases toxins back into the bloodstream and causes illness. The use of bentonite clay in cleaning the digestive tract is a traditional practice in many cultures and has been used for thousands of years as both an internal and external purification aid.

Bentonite clay's negatively charged and large rectangular surface attracts and captures positively charged toxins and waste many times its own weight. Think of bentonite clay as a sticky sponge that can soak up waste lining the intestine. It attaches to and pulls waste out of the pouches so it can be removed from the body. This is a relatively quick process I did over three days, which resulted in me losing several pounds of waste from my colon. I felt really light, energized, and my body rejected certain unhealthy foods like processed bread for a period of time.

Psyllium husk is a natural dietary fiber used to promote excretion of the bentonite clay and its trapped waste.[174] Psyllium husk is a soluble fiber used primarily as a gentle, bulk-forming laxative. Psyllium comes from a shrub-like herb called *Plantago ovata* that is common to India and grows less commonly in other parts of the world. Psyllium husk has been used to relieve both constipation and diarrhea and has been used to treat other intestinal problems like irritable bowel syndrome and hemorrhoids.

I performed the cleanse over a three-day period and was able to pull a lot of the waste out of the colon in a short time, but not all of it. Eating a plant based diet and taking herbs for three months was able to deepen the clean, while producing no detox symptoms. I used a bentonite clay and psyllium husk cleansing kit by ariseandshine.com that I found to be really helpful as a jump-starter for the long-term herbal cleanse. The specific kit also uses some of the herbs that are part of Dr. Sebi's herbal products, like cascara sagrada, ginger and rhubarb root.

Kidney Cleanse

The simplest kidney cleanse involves drinking the required amount of water the body needs to remain properly hydrated. The Institute of Medicine set the general daily recommendation for total water from beverages and food for men at approximately 3.7 liters (125 ounces daily) of total water, and for women approximately 2.7 liters (91 ounces.[175] The upper limit for water consumption was not set. Dr. Sebi recommended one gallon of water a day while taking diuretic herbs, and that was the amount of water I drank while taking herbs. It remains the amount of water I drink today.

Drinking enough water is essential in flushing and cleaning the kidneys. When there isn't enough water in the body, waste flowing through the kidneys becomes concentrated. The concentrated waste damages the kidneys and reduces their ability to properly filter waste. Drinking the recommended amount of water reduces the concentration of waste. This reduces the strain put on the kidneys and gives them a rest so energy can be put towards healing.

A watermelon cleanse has been used to dissolve and remove kidney stones. The watermelon cleanse is simple and calls for eating one whole seeded watermelon in one day, while drinking the recommended amount of water. The watermelon cleanse is not recommended for use by people who have diabetes. The three month herbal cleanse also addresses cleaning and strengthening the kidneys but this is done over an extended period of time. The water and watermelon cleanse can be used to make the herbal cleaning process easier and more effective.

Small-Intestine Cleanse

I discovered the consumption of dairy and its inflammation causing casein protein was a major reason for the over production of mucus in the body. Combine this with the factory farming processes that introduce unnatural growth hormones and disease into dairy products, its harm is multiplied. This inflammatory response to the consumption of the pathogens and toxins in dairy can lead to the development of a harmful mucoid layer in the small intestine that can interfere with the absorption of nutrients through it into the bloodstream. The mucoid layer can become very difficult to remove because proteins, pathogens, and toxins become stuck in it and ordinary measures won't remove it.

I discovered the harmful mucoid layer in the small intestine had to be addressed in two steps.[176, 177] The proteins stuck in the mucoid layer had to be dissolved first, so the mucoid layer could be broken down and removed. I used the plant-based bromelain and papain enzymes to dissolve the proteins, and mullein to dissolve the harmful mucoid layer.

85

The small intestine constantly produces its own mucus to protect the lining of the small intestine from the partially digested food that moves into it from the stomach. Removing the harmful mucoid layer allows for the production of healthy mucus to line the intestinal wall, which allows also for the free movement of nutrients through its wall into the bloodstream.

Bromelain is extracted from pineapples and is a mixture of protein-digesting enzymes called proteolytic enzymes. Pineapples contain two main protein-digesting enzymes, one found in the stem, and the other in the fruit. Stem bromelain is the more common source of bromelain. Pineapple has a long history of traditional use among the people native to Central and South America. They have used pineapple dressings to reduce inflammation in wounds and skin injuries, and drank pineapple juice to treat indigestion. Papain's use has been similar to the use of bromelain. Papaya's papain enzyme is an antiseptic and anti-inflammatory and has been used to treat burns, bedsores, skin ulcers, and wounds, and to remove dead skin. Both have been used as meat tenderizers because of their protein-digesting properties.

I used mullein to remove the mucoid layer once the trapped proteins were dissolved. The mullein plant is native to northern Africa, Asia, and Europe, and was brought to the Americas and Australia. Mullein was known by many different names: Aaron's rod, Adam's flannel, Indian tobacco, Jacob's staff, Jupiter's staff, Peter's staff, blanket leaf, bullock's lungwort, cow's lungwort, feltwort, hare's beard, lady's foxglove, mullein leaf, and many more. Its many names are an indication of how popular and effective the herb was. Many of the names are derived from the velvety texture of its big mullein leaf. The lungwort identification is associated with mullein leaf's traditional use as a treatment for relieving cough and congestion. Mullein leaf has long been used as an expectorant for treating respiratory congestion because it promotes the ejection of mucus from the lungs. My research of mullein led me to use it to specially target the small intestine, though it would also help remove excess mucus from other areas of the body.

The change in the makeup of my stool was an indication of the herbs effectiveness. When I first adopted the plant-based diet, the stool was flaky, which indicated to me that the food wasn't being digested as efficiently as it could be. Taking the herbs gradually led to the stool losing its flakiness and having a more cohesive composition. My energy also increased another level, which indicated more nutrients were being absorbed into the bloodstream.

Liver-and-Gallbladder Cleanse

The liver screens the blood for toxins, viruses, and bacteria. It detoxifies alcohol and other synthetic drugs and plays a major part in the supporting the body's immune system. The liver produces Kupffer cells, a type of white-blood-cell macrophage, to destroy viruses, bacteria, old blood cells, and other substances being filtered through the liver.[178] When the liver is damaged, its ability to fight infection, manufacture essential enzymes and proteins, secrete bile to aid digestion, absorb and store vitamins A, D, E, and K, manufacture and regulate hormones, and remove waste from the blood is compromised.

Recreational and prescription drugs and toxins absorbed into the body through the skin, breathing, or by the ingestion of toxin containing foods, all damage the liver in high concentrations. Autoimmune diseases and cancer also damage the liver.[179, 180]

A damaged liver can present with the following symptoms:

- Fatigue, lack of appetite, loss of energy, weakness, weight loss and nausea
- Jaundice: The liver can't remove bilirubin from the blood, which causes a yellowing of the skin and the white part of the eyes
- Nails become curved and white rather than pink
- Digestion problems resulting in a loss of appetite, weight loss, and anemia
- Lighter stool due to the lack of bile production

- Blood clotting takes longer because the liver's ability to make the clotting protein, fibrinogen, is compromised
- The body retains water and becomes bloated because its ability to help the kidneys remove water is compromised

Burdock root, dandelion root, yellow dock, and sarsaparilla have been used by cultures all over the world for centuries to strengthen and clean the liver.[181, 182, 183, 184, 185] Their phytonutrients stimulate the immune system and cell repair. I wanted to do all I could to quicken the cleansing and repair of my liver and through research I found out a compromised gallbladder could put pressure on the liver and compromise its functioning. I decided to do a short-term and unconventional gallbladder cleanse that would aid the proper functioning of the liver. I performed short-term gallbladder cleanse designed by Dr. Hulda Clark's as a jump-starter to promote a quicker and more effective long-term deep cleanse of the liver through the use of herbs.

The gallbladder cleanse is a one day cleanse that focused on removing gallstones and waste from the gallbladder. This would take pressure off the liver by allowing the proper and unobstructed delivery of bile from the liver to the gallbladder. The cleanse is unconventional because it relies on the consumption of Epsom salt to relax the bile ducts so gallstones can move freely through the bile ducts. This cleanse should not be done by people who can't tolerate Epsom salt. The one day cleanse also involves consuming apple juice and its malic acid, which dissolves the cohesion between gallstones. Coconut oil is consumed to stimulate the gallbladder to contract to move out gallstones. The original recipe called for the use of lemons or grapefruits to cut the taste of the oil to make it easier to swallow. Key limes can be used instead since they are alkaline, or they don't have to be used at all.

There is some risk in doing the cleanse because you would be purposely trying to dislodge gallstones from the gallbladder and move them through the ducts. There is the possibility they could get stuck in the ducts, but the possibility would still exist without doing the cleanse.

At least with me doing the cleanse I purposefully relaxed the ducts so the gallstones could move through freely, instead of waiting on a ticking time bomb and have the gallstones build up and block the ducts. I decided to take the risk, but I was also assured by the many people who did the cleanse and showed pictures of the stones they passed. I hadn't found one testimony where a person ran into an issue passing gallstones. Doing the one day cleanse I successfully passed many gallstones. For more information on the cleanse please visit this link: http://www.naturallifeenergy.com/liver-gallbladder-cleanse/.[186]

MY PLANT-BASED DIET

My plant-based diet is an 80/10/10 diet consisting of roughly 80 percent carbohydrates, 10 percent fat, and 10 percent protein. A well-rounded plant-based or plant-centered diet naturally consists of this ratio of nutrients, which is perfectly suited to optimally support health.

My diet has evolved to consist of a high concentration of fruits, but when I first adopted a plant-based diet, it consisted of a higher concentration of vegetables. The transition to a diet consisting largely of fruits was a natural transition and a logical one. When I first adopted a plant-based diet, I carried excess weight, which meant I carried extra stored energy (glycogen and fat) and waste in my intestines. In order to use up my stored energy and remove the waste in my intestines I focused on consuming vegetables because they were concentrated with fiber and micronutrients. Micronutrients consist of vitamins, minerals, and phytonutrients. In contrast to vegetables, fruits contain more macronutrients, which is energy and in this case are carbohydrates.

The micronutrients from the vegetables provided more vitamins and minerals to strengthen my organs, and build and repair cells. The phytonutrients supported my immune system, and fiber strengthened and cleaned my digestive tract by supporting proper muscle function to remove toxic built-up waste. A crucial part of my approach to the plant-based diet was drinking a lot of blended vegetable juice, which allowed me to consume much more vegetables that if I had eaten them whole. This allowed me to super saturate my body with micronutrients which greatly assisted my healing process.

For energy I decided to snack on almonds. The almonds satisfied my need for eating something whole and something I could crunch on. Almonds compared to other nuts like walnuts, contain more fiber and less fat. Though I chose to focus of getting a lot of my energy from natural sources of fat like almonds, my weight dropped around thirty pounds and I have kept the weight off easily even after years of adopting a whole food plant based diet.

THE PROCESS

I ate five to six small meals a day, made up of food on the nutritional guide, and each meal was around two hours apart. My meals during my transition to a plant-based diet and during the herbal cleanse consisted mostly of vegetable juice, nuts, salads, and water. Through studying the foods on the nutritional list, I grouped together several foods I felt best complemented each other to make the vegetable juice. The vegetable juice consisted of kale, cilantro, ginger, cayenne pepper, flax seed, apple, and water. It took on a life of its own, becoming known as the "Bam Bam" juice (see recipes). I used to make it with hemp seed when I was concerned about consuming enough protein, but as I became more comfortable with the merits of the diet, I realized I didn't need the extra protein.

Birth of the "Bam Bam" Juice

Kale is one of the most nutrient-dense leafy greens, and it boosts the immune system.[187, 188] Cilantro is an excellent heavy-metal detoxifier.[189, 190] Ginger has antibacterial properties, reduces chronic inflammation, reduces high blood pressure, soothes the stomach, and helps build good gut bacteria.[191, 192] Cayenne pepper prevents LDL cholesterol oxidation, lowers blood pressure, reduces pain in the body, assists weight loss, and fights irritable bowel syndrome.[193, 194, 195] Flax seed is high in omega-3 that provides energy, is anti-inflammatory, and helps to keep the brain healthy.[196]

I generally don't mix vegetables and fruits together because I find it can cause indigestion. I do use an apple in my vegetable juice because it mixes well with vegetables without causing digestion issues. I use an apple in the vegetable juice for two reasons. The iron in vegetables is the non-heme form of iron that is not easily absorbed into the body. Vitamin C allows the body to easily absorb the non-heme iron and the apple supplies vitamin C.[197, 198] The addition of the apple also adds texture and some sweetness to the vegetable juice. Adding water to the blended produce is helpful. The body also is made up from 50 up to 75 percent water,[199] so it is important to keep the body properly hydrated. Dehydration can lead to weakness, dizziness, confusion, and fatigue.[200]

The "Bam Bam" juice is also high in fiber that supports the health of the digestive tract and feeds the good bacteria in the body. I blended the vegetables instead of using a juicer to juice them so I would maintain all of the nutrients of the whole food. Blending the vegetables makes it easier for the body to digest them and also allowed me to consume far more vegetables than if I were to eat them whole. This allowed me to flood my body with nutrients to speed the cleaning and healing process.

Meal Plan

1st meal: Early morning—After waking up, drink two 16-ounce glasses of Bam Bam juice and cleansing herbs.

2nd meal: 9:00–11:00 a.m.—28-ounce bottle of "Bam Bam."

3rd meal: 11:00–1:00 p.m.—Drink 28-ounce bottle of water and snack on almonds.

4th meal: 1:00–3:00 p.m.—Drink 28-ounce bottle of water and cleansing herbs. Nice salad (mixed greens, chickpeas, onions, tomatoes, cucumbers, and hummus).

5th meal: 7:00 p.m. dinner—Cup a cooked quinoa with steamed zucchini and sautéed mushrooms, or a quinoa salad. Water. Snack on almonds or walnuts if needed.

I took my herbs 2-3 times daily for 3 months, along with following this regimen. I never felt lethargic or hungry. Eating small, light, whole-food meals didn't overwhelm my digestive system. It allowed the food to digest quickly and provided a steady flow of energy and nutrients. My digestive system became incredibly efficient, which required having a bathroom nearby.

CHAPTER 16:

LEARNING TO EAT FOR HEALTH FIRST

We need to change our paradigm about how we think of food from one that is centered on "living to eat" to one that is centered on "eating to live." We need to change our paradigm from looking at allopathic or pharmacological medicine as our cure for disease, to start looking at natural plant life and herbs and their nutrients and phytonutrients as our defense against disease and our means to reverse disease. We need to saturate our bodies with uncompromised nutrients and phytonutrients, which is best achieved by eating diets centered on eating non-hybrid raw plant foods. This means eating diets centered on eating fruits and vegetables, supplemented with legumes, nuts, seeds, and whole grains. The foods on the nutritional guide are more supportive of health because the guide avoids plant foods that are highly hybridized with compromised nutritional structures.

The nutritional guide avoids highly starchy foods that slow digestion and compromise the balance of flora (immune system bacteria). Foods on the guide contain high levels of good resistant starch, like quinoa, which is not digested but travels to the colon where it feeds the good bacteria. The good bacteria feed on the resistant starch and produces a short-chain fatty-acid called butyrate. Butyrate is the fuel source that feeds the cells that line and protect the colon. Without the butyrate to feed and strengthen the cells lining the colon, the colon can become inflamed, start bleeding, and deteriorate. It is very important to keep the colon healthy because 80% of the immune system is in the digestive tract, and a large amount of it is concentrated in the colon.

Hybridization has produced many foods that are high in amylose and amylopectin starch. These starches are digested, unlike resistant starch, and are digested slowly because they have very complex molecular structures. These starches, found greatly concentrated in high starchy foods like white potatoes, compromise the digestive tract and its immune system. These starches are difficult to digest and don't provide quick burning energy to support cell and muscle function like carbohydrates in fruits do. They also bind with nutrients making them less bioavailable, and their digestion produces byproducts that compromise the natural balance of the flora or good bacteria in the digestive tract.

We are living in a very toxic environment and we need to saturate the body with foods that support health and the immune system, while introducing the least amount of substances that compromise it. We have less control over the toxins in the environment we breathe in and touch, but we have much more control of the toxins and pathogens we introduce into our bodies through the food and drink we consume. It has been established the meat, dairy, and processed foods introduce the most pathogens and toxins into the body that compromise health. Natural non-hybrid plant foods are better to consume because they are saturated with vitamins, minerals, and phytonutrients that strengthen organs and fights disease.

Consuming raw foods generally is the best way to saturate your body with vitamins, minerals, and phytonutrients. An important thing to remember is you have to chew raw foods like leafy greens very well to make more of their nutrients bioavailable. Just because plant foods contain a lot of nutrients, that doesn't necessarily mean they are bioavailable. Nutrients are bioavailable when during digestion the nutrients can actually be extracted from the cells of the plants and absorbed into the bloodstream. This is why I advocate highly for drinking blended vegetable juices and fruit smoothies.

Blenders break down the cell walls of plant food much more efficiently than chewing does. This allows for much more of the plant's nutrients to be actually utilized by the body. To best support health we should drink a lot of blended vegetables and fruit smoothies throughout the day. If you are newly transitioning to a plant based diet it is better to concentrate on consuming more blended vegetables. The reason for this is vegetables are more micronutrient dense than fruits. Vegetables contain less energy than fruits, and consuming less energy will allow the body to use up stored energy and release toxins that are stored along with them so they can be removed from the body. The greater concentration of fiber found in leafy greens and their phytonutrients will provide greater assistance in removing toxins from the body. I know we don't want to live by juice alone, so eating hearty salads to supplement the vegetables juices is a good way to focus on fiber and micronutrient consumption, while satisfying the need to chew on something.

The next way best to maximize your nutrient consumption is to eat steamed plant foods. You can use steaming pots, or add plant foods to a pan or pot, add some water and heat the food on a low fire. The low heat will help to keep the foods raw, by keeping most of the foods enzymes and nutrients intact, while softening the cell walls so the nutrients become more bioavailable. Some nutrients are water soluble, like vitamin C and many B vitamins, and will leech into the water. It is better to not waste the water and drink it. Boiling plant foods like butternut squash will make more of its nutrients bioavailable, but boiling will pull water soluble vitamins out of the butternut squash. It is better to make soups out of butternut squash, or at least drink the cooled water than remains after boiling the squash.

Heating food by frying or baking at high temperatures causes the most damage to the enzymes and nutrients of plant foods. Frying and baking foods above 248 degrees Fahrenheit can cause certain sugars or carbohydrates to turn into toxic compounds called acrylamides, which support cancer development and proliferation. The formation of acrylamides has not been found with steaming or boiling. Oils are commonly used when frying and baking. Excessive oil consumption is associated impaired endothelium function in arteries.

Arteries contain a layer of cells called the endothelium. The endothelium controls the artery's ability to dilate and constrict to move blood and nutrients on their way. The endothelium is the body's largest endocrine or hormone producing organ in the body. It regulates vascular cell growth, clotting and thinning of blood, inflammatory processes, and artery permeability. The excessive consumption of oils compromises the endothelium, but not the consumption of these fats in their natural form, as in olives and not olive oil. Oils have been removed from the fiber and nutrients they were originally wrapped with, which controlled the digestion of the fat. Oils are not packaged with these regulators and this undermines their normal and proper digestion, which compromises arterial and heart function.

CHAPTER 17:

RECIPES

The focus of these recipes is to optimally support health and a healthy transition to a plant-based diet. The focus is on raw foods especially on vegetable and fruit smoothie recipes.

WATER

Water is arguably the must underappreciated and under utilized nutrient which holds hunger at bay. Most people are dehydrated to some level, which is major reason for the proliferation of disease. The body is made up of around 70% water and all of the cells of the body need to be adequately hydrated to support proper metabolic function. In general, we should consume 1 gallon of water a day to support the optimal health of cells.

Ingredients:
1 gallon of spring water

It is arguably best to drink spring water because it is natural, or the most natural water. Bottled spring water does undergo minimal filtration to remove impurities. We live in highly industrialized societies that produces toxins that end up in the water supply. Spring water is minimally filtered to remove these toxins, but small amounts of environmental contaminants are not completely filtered. Water is essential for healthy living so we should not reduce our water consumption, even though water sources are being compromised by industrial pollution. Developing a strong immune system by eating plants and their nutrients and phytonutrients will go a long way in neutralizing these toxins.

Some people choose to bypass the issue of residual toxins being in bottled spring water by drinking distilled water. Distilled water removes everything besides the water, both good and bad. There is a natural balance of minerals in spring water that buffers the water's pH, and removing the minerals leaves the water open to becoming acidic. The good thing about distilled water is that is doesn't contain harmful industrial pollutants, the bad thing is there also nothing in it to stop the growth of bad bacteria and to keep the water's pH from becoming acidic. If you decide to drink bottled distilled water uncap and cap the bottle as quick as possible to reduce the amount of pathogens, toxins, and air getting into the water. It is also good to store bottles that have been opened in the fridge to slow the growth of microbes.

Some people opt to use tap water purifiers to purify tap water, or ionizers to purify and to add minerals back to the tap water to alkalize and raise the water's pH. Drinking straight tap water should be avoided, regardless of where you live. Some places or municipality's water contains less chemicals than others, but they all use synthetic chemicals like chlorine to kill pathogens in the water. These chemicals attack the body, throw off homeostasis, and weaken the immune system. Some municipalities add fluoride, which has been seen in studies to lower IQ, especially in growing children.

JUICES AND SMOOTHIES

Method
A blender, preferably a high speed blender, is used to make all vegetable juices and fruit smoothies. Water is added to the juices and smoothies to make them more easily drinkable. You can use more or

less water depending on the consistency of the juice or smoothie you want.

Rinse your produce thoroughly to remove residual surface pesticides and contamination.

Cut the Food Stickers Off
The produce we purchase have stickers on them to identify what they are. The glue on these stickers is carcinogenic so instead of peeling off the sticker and washing the area, cut that piece of skin off and discard it because remnants of the glue will likely remain on the skin.

Removing the Skin from Fruits?
The concern with eating the skin of vegetables and fruits is the use of pesticides. It is important to know that vitamins, minerals and nutrients are concentrated in the skin. Plants use the nutrients to grow and to protect themselves from the environment, and the first line of defense is the skin.
It is better to eat organic produce because the use of harmful synthetic fertilizer is reduced. Whether using organic or conventional produce it is good to thoroughly rinse the produce to remove residual surface pesticides and contamination from handling. Though eating organic produce is better than eating conventional produce, eating conventional produce is better than eating the harmful pathogens and toxins in meat, dairy, and processed foods, because produce contains health protecting phytonutrients and nutrients.

Blending Vegetables and Fruits and Usage
It is better to drink the vegetable juices and fruit smoothies as soon as you make them. Blending vegetables and fruits breaks apart their cell walls, allowing the trapped nutrients to become bioavailable. This also leaves them susceptible to oxidation, which is why is it better to drink them right away. If you don't drink them right away, it is best to drink the juices or smoothies within the day you make them. Store the juices and smoothies in closed containers in the fridge to slow oxidation. You can travel with the juices and smoothies, and it is better to use bottles with air tight lids. The longer you go without drinking the juices or smoothies the more time you are giving the nutrients in the juices to degrade. It is better to use glass or stainless steel containers instead of

plastic containers to avoid chemicals leeching from plastic containers into the juice or smoothie. I travel with my juices and smoothies daily in stainless steel bottles.

"Bam Bam Juice"

Makes 64 oz. of juice. The "Bam Bam" juice is dense in micronutrients, detoxifies heavy metals, reduces chronic inflammation and high blood pressure, sooths the stomach and builds good gut bacteria, prevents LDL cholesterol oxidation, reduces body pain, assists weight loss, fights irritable bowel syndrome, has antibacterial properties, and supports the immune system.

Ingredients:
4 cup kale (loosely chopped)
5 stems of cilantro
1 apple
1-inch piece of ginger root
⅛ - ¼ tsp cayenne pepper
1 tbsp of organic flax seed
28fl oz. water

Directions:
Add all the ingredients together and blend to your desired consistency. Add enough water afterwards to make 64 oz. of juice. This makes 4 16 oz. glasses of "Bam Bam" juice. I drink 2 16 oz. glasses first thing in the morning, and I bottle the rest and drink it a little later for my work day breakfast. The juice is not sweet, tastes like vegetables, and may take a little time to get used to. Just think of it as your natural medicine and just drink it down.

BerLime (Juice)

Ingredients:
1 cucumber

juice of 1 key lime
Add enough water to the blender jar to make 32 oz. of juice.

Directions:
Cut up the cucumber with or without skin into to several pieces to make easier to blend. Either squeeze the juice from the lime or scoop out the interior of the lime. Blend to desired consistency.

Nutrients are concentrated in the skin of the cucumber and it is better to consume the skin to get all it phytonutrients and health protecting properties. It is better to use organic when intending to consume the skin because the use of synthetic pesticides is avoided. Rinse thoroughly. If you are using conventional produce rinse thoroughly to remove surface pesticides and contamination. The juice will be more fibrous using the cucumber skin than blending the cucumber without the skin.

GinApple (Juice)

Ingredients:
2 apples
1-inch piece of ginger root
3 pitted dates
Add enough water to the blender jar to make 32 oz. of juice. Add more water for thinner juice.

Directions:
The skin of the ginger contains nutrients. Use a coarse brush to remove dirt from the ginger. Cut the ginger in smaller pieces to make it easier to blend. Blend to your desired consistency, and add more water if needed.

Nice and Dandy (Juice)

Ingredients:
2 cup of loosely chopped dandelion leaves
½ apple
½ cucumber
½ inch piece of ginger root
⅛ tsp of cayenne pepper
Add enough water to the blender jar to make 32 oz. of juice. Add more water for thinner juice.

Calla Loo Loo (Smoothie)

I don't usually mix vegetables with fruits other than an apple to avoid digestion issues like gas. For those who aren't bothered by mixing vegetables and fruits this is a smoother tasting vegetable drink.

Ingredients:
2 cups of loosely chopped callaloo leaves
1 banana
½ apple
½ inch of ginger root
Add enough water to the blender jar to make 32 oz. of juice. Add more water for thinner juice.

Spicy Loo Loo (Juice)

Ingredients:
2 cups of loosely chopped callaloo leaves
½ cucumber
½ apple
½ inch of ginger root
⅛ tsp cayenne pepper
Add enough water to the blender jar to make 32 oz. of juice. Add more water for thinner juice.

Sweet Dream Strawberry (Smoothie)

Ingredients:
5 Strawberries
3 pitted dates
2 bananas

Add enough water to the blender jar to make 32 oz. of juice. Add more water for thinner juice.

Sweet and Tangy (Smoothie)

Ingredients:
3 pitted dates
2 bananas
juice of 1 key lime
Add enough water to the blender jar to make 32 oz. of juice. Add more water for thinner juice.

Sticky Prickly (Smoothie)

Ingredients:
1-inch slice of nopales prickly pear cactus paddle (thorns removed)
3 pitted dates
1 banana
1 cup of coconut water
Add enough water to the blender jar to make 32 oz. of juice. Add more water for thinner juice.

You can find nopales paddles Spanish and Caribbean supermarkets and grocery stores. Nopales is used to support weight loss, improve skin health, improve digestion, boost the immune system, and optimize metabolic activity.

Goji Berry Tart (Smoothie)

Ingredients:
¼ cup of dried goji berries
2 bananas
3 tbsp coconut milk
⅓ of hemp seeds
juice of 1 key lime
Add enough water to the blender jar to make 32 oz. of juice. Add more water for thinner juice. Goji berries are highly antioxidant.

Tamarind Tart (Juice)

Ingredients:
⅛ cup of tamarind pulp
3 pitted dates
Add enough water to the blender jar to make 32 oz. of juice. Add more water for thinner juice. You eat either by the whole tamarind and remove the tamarind, or you can buy tamarind pulp by itself in packages for Caribbean grocery stores. Tamarind is a great detoxifier of fluoride.

Strawberry Sour (Juice)

Ingredients:
5 Strawberries
¼ cup of frozen soursop or fresh soursop pulp. (Fresh soursop can be difficult to find. Goya sells a frozen soursop package that consists of only soursop pulp. You can find it in the frozen section in Spanish supermarkets and grocery stores.)
3 pitted dates
Add enough water to the blender jar to make 32 oz. of juice. Add more water for thinner juice.

M8 Spicy (Juice)

Ingredients:
2 cups of loosely chopped mustard greens
2 plum tomatoes
½ cucumber
⅛ tsp of cayenne pepper
¼ red bell pepper
Add enough water to the blender jar to make 32 oz. of juice. Add more water for thinner juice.

Ginger Revival (Juice)

Ingredients:
1-inch piece of ginger root
2 plum tomatoes
½ cucumber
⅛ tsp of cayenne pepper
¼ red bell pepper
Add enough water to the blender jar to make 32 oz. of juice. Add more water for thinner juice. Ginger is great for soothing the stomach and reducing nausea.

FOOD DISHES

Quinoa

Serves 2-4
Ingredients:
1 cup quinoa
3 scallions (chopped)
¼ green bell pepper (chopped)
½ plum tomato (chopped)
1 ½ cups water
¼ tsp coconut oil
¼ tsp sea salt
⅛ tsp thyme
dash of cayenne pepper

Directions:
1. Soak the quinoa for at least 5 minutes, then rinse and strain.
2. Add all the ingredients to a saucepan and bring to a boil.
3. Reduce the fire and let simmer for 15 minutes until the water is absorbed.

Vegetable Stuffed Quinoa with Steamed Zucchini

Serves 2-4
Ingredients:
1 cup quinoa
1 ½ cups water
2 tbsp coconut milk
¾ cup mushrooms (chopped)
1-inch section red bell pepper (chopped)
¼ onion (chopped)

1 plum tomato (chopped)
½ tsp sea salt
spices: dash of basil, oregano, thyme, red pepper flakes

⅓ zucchini (sliced)

Directions:
1. Soak the quinoa for at least 5 minutes, then rinse and strain.
2. Add all the ingredients (except for the zucchini) to a saucepan and bring to a boil.
3. Reduce the fire and let simmer for 15 minutes until the water is absorbed.
4. Steam the zucchini slices in a steamer for 5-10 minutes.
5. Plate and serve

Stuffed Bell Peppers

Serves 1-2
Ingredients:
1 cup of quinoa
1 ½ cups water
2 green bell peppers
1 lb. oyster or other mushroom
1 tbsp (grape-seed or coconut or avocado oil)
½ red bell peppers chopped fine
½ tsp basil
½ tsp dill
½ tsp sea salt
⅛ tsp of cayenne pepper

Directions:
1. Soak quinoa for 5-10 minutes and rinse. Combine quinoa and water in a saucepan. Bring to a boil than reduce to a medium low flame and cook for 15-20 minutes. Set aside.

2. Remove stem, cut off tops, and hollow out the green bell peppers. Steam in a steamer until softened.

3. Sauté mushrooms in oil over medium heat. It is important to not cook on high heat to maintain the integrity of the oil and food. Remove mushrooms from pan at let cool.

4. Combine cooked quinoa, mushrooms, and spices and mix.

5. Stuff green bell peppers with e quinoa mix and serve.

Optional:

6. You can bake the stuffed quinoa in an oven preheated to 250 degrees for 15 minutes.

Seasoned Wild Rice

Serves 1-2

Ingredients:

1 cup wild rice (soak wild rice overnight)

2-3 cups water (3 cups of water is you didn't soak the rice overnight)

1 tbsp coconut oil

2 tsp oregano

½ tsp sea salt

⅛ tsp cayenne pepper

2-3 scallions (chopped)

1 plum tomato (chopped)

Directions:

Soaking the rice in water over night reduces the cooking time for the rice.

Add all of the ingredients to a saucepan over a high heat and let come to a boil. Cover saucepan and reduce to a simmer and allow the water to absorb into the rice. If you soaked the rice overnight cook the rice for 25 minutes. If you did not soak the rice overnight, cook for 50-60 minutes.

Roasted Large Cap Portobello Mushrooms and Yellow Squash

Serves 1-2
Ingredients:
3 large Portobello mushrooms
9 – ½ inch slices of yellow squash
avocado oil (brush on front and back of mushrooms)
½ lime
spice (coriander, cayenne pepper, oregano, sea salt)

Directions:
1. Pull off the Portobello mushroom stems and scoop out the fins with a spoon.
2. Brush on avocado oil on the front and back of the mushrooms.
3. Squeeze a little lime over the tops of the mushrooms.
4. Sprinkle on the spices on the mushrooms and yellow squash but keep the mushrooms and squash separate.
5. Heat oven to 400 degrees Fahrenheit.
6. Place mushrooms on roasting pan, scooped out side facing up. Cook for 10 minutes.
7. Carefully remove the pan and mushrooms, and add 3 seasoned yellow squash slices to each mushroom top. Put roasting pan back into the oven.
8. Cook the mushrooms and squash for another 10 minutes.
9. Remove from oven and serve hot.

Spelt Spaghetti

Serves 2-3
Ingredients:
1 – 8 oz. box of Spelt Spaghetti (Nature's Legacy makes a product that is only made from spelt and water.)

Directions:
1. Boil 2 quarts of water in pot.
2. Slowly add in the spelt spaghetti. (I like to break the spaghetti into thirds to make it easier to eat.)
3. Cook for 10 minutes, stirring occasionally. Don't overcook.
4. Drain and plate. (Goes great with the butternut squash plum tomato sauce.)

Butternut Squash Plum Tomato Spaghetti Sauce

Ingredients:
½ butternut squash (remove skin and cut into cubes)
¼ plum tomato (chopped)
1 cup water
spices: dash of cayenne pepper, onion, basil, bay leaf, oregano, thyme, savory, coriander, and salt

Directions:
1. Add butternut squash cubes to pot, cover with water and boil until squash becomes tender. Remove squash from water.
2. Add squash, tomato, and spices to a blender and blend, slowly add water until you reach desired consistency.
3. Add to a container, let cool, and refrigerate.

Simply Chayote Squash

Serves 1
Ingredients:
1 chayote squash
¼ teaspoon of coconut oil
dash cayenne pepper
dash of sea salt

Directions:
Serves as a light snack or part of a dish
1. Wash and cut chayote squash in half. The seed can by eaten and it has a nice texture.
2. Add chayote, oil, and enough water to cover the chayote in a saucepan. Boil for 20 minutes until fork can penetrate the squash, but the squash should still maintain some firmness.
3. Remove form water. Season with cayenne pepper and sea salt to taste.

Vegetable Medley Sauté

Serves 4
Ingredients:
1 cup mushrooms (sliced)
1 zucchini (sliced)
1 yellow squash (sliced)
1 red pepper (chopped)
1 green pepper (chopped)
2 plum tomatoes (chopped)
½ red onion (finely chopped)
½ cup chayote (finely chopped)
3 tbsp grape-seed oil or avocado oil (they are higher smoking points and can withstand heat better)

⅛ tsp cayenne pepper
⅛ tsp sea salt

Directions:
1. Add oil to a saucepan on medium heat. Let the oil get hot.
2. Add in mushrooms and onions and sauté for 4 minutes.
3. Add in the rest of the vegetables and spices and sauté for 8-10 minutes.

SOUPS

Chickpea Butternut Squash Soup

Serves 2
Ingredients:
15 oz. cooked chickpeas
1 ½ section of a butternut squash
¼ plum tomato
¼ cup coconut milk
1 cup water (add more water to make thinner soup)
pinch of dill
pinch of all spice
pinch of cayenne pepper
⅛ tsp of sea salt

Directions:
Add all of the ingredients to a blender and blend to your desired consistency. Add the blended ingredients to a saucepan over a medium/high flame until it starts to boil or air bubbles rise. Reduce the flame to medium low and cook for 30 minutes.

Butternut Squash Ginger Soup

Serves 2
Ingredients:
1 section of a butternut squash
¼ cup coconut milk
1 tbsp coconut oil
3 cups water (add more water to make thinner soup)
2 tsp minced fresh ginger
1 tbsp date sugar
½ cup of diced onions

1 tsp finely chopped fresh thyme
⅛ tsp of sea salt
pinch of all spice
pinch of cayenne pepper

Directions:
1. Remove skin and seeds from butternut squash, and cut squash into medium sized cubes.
2. Add cubes to saucepan and cover cubes with water. Boil until squash becomes soft.
3. Remove softened squash from water and discard water.
4. Add butternut squash, coconut milk, and coconut oil to the blender and blend until smooth. Add in the rest of the ingredients and 1 cup of water and blend for a few seconds.
5. Transfer mix to saucepan and stir in the remaining 2 cups of water to the desired consistency. Add more water if wanted.
6. Bring to a boil, reduce heat and let simmer for for 15 minutes.

Cream of Avocado Mushroom Soup

Serves 2-4
Ingredients:
2 avocados (scoop out flesh and discard skin)
juice of 1 key lime
2 cups hot water
⅛ tsp of cayenne pepper
⅛ tsp of sea salt
dash of all spice

1 tbsp coconut oil or grape seed oil
1 cup of sliced mushrooms
1 red bell pepper (diced)
¼ yellow onion (finely chopped)
3 plum tomatoes (diced)

3 sprigs of fresh thyme leaves

Directions:
1. Add hot water, avocados, lime juice, cayenne pepper, sea salt, and all spice in a blender. Pulse until smooth.
2. Heat oil in saucepan over medium and stir in mushrooms, red bell pepper, onion, tomatoes, and thyme until they become soft.
3. Add in avocado mix to the saucepan and simmer for 5 minutes.

SALADS

Kale, Mushroom, Walnut, Avocado Salad

Serves 2-3
Ingredients:
6 Lacinato kale leaves (chopped)
10 crushed walnuts
¼ onion (diced)
¼ red bell pepper (diced)
½ plum tomato (sliced)
20 mushrooms slices
½ - 1 tbsp avocado oil

Dressing:
1 tbsp key lime juice
1 tbsp sesame oil
1 plum tomato
⅛ tsp of sea salt
¼ avocado

Directions:
1. Dressing: Blend the lime juice, sesame oil, plum tomato, salt, and avocado together until smooth.
2. Sauté the mushrooms in the avocado oil. Let cool afterwards.
3. Mix the the kale, walnuts, onion, pepper, tomato, and mushrooms together.
4. Add your desired amount of dressing to the salad and massage into the salad until until the dressing evenly coats the entire salad.
(This salad should be used as a treat because you want to minimize your use of oils, and this recipe calls for the use of oil.)

Chickpea Salad

Serves 2-3
Ingredients:
1 – 15 oz. can of chickpeas or 15 oz. of cooked chickpeas (cold)
¼ red onion (chopped)
1-2 plum tomatoes (chopped)
¼ red bell pepper (chopped)
¼ green bell pepper (chopped)
1 tbsp key lime juice
1 tbsp coconut oil
⅛ tsp of cayenne pepper
dash of cilantro
sea salt (optional)

Directions:
1. Add all the ingredient to a bowl mix and toss thoroughly.

Quinoa and Chickpea Salad

Serves 2-3
Ingredients:
1 cup quinoa
1 ½ cups water
¼ tsp coconut oil

4 oz. cooked chickpeas
¼ cup red onion (diced)
¼ green bell pepper (chopped)
⅛ tsp of cayenne pepper
½ tbsp of coconut oil
sea salt (optional)

Directions:

1. Add quinoa, water, and ¼ tsp coconut oil to saucepan. Let boil and reduce heat to simmer. Simmer for 15 minutes until water is absorbed.

2. Remove quinoa from fire and let cool.

3. Add cooked chickpeas, onion, bell pepper, cayenne pepper, and ½ tsp of coconut oil to a bowl and mix. Stir in cold quinoa.

Mix Mix Alkaline Veggie Salad

Serves 2

Ingredients:

15 kale leaves (chopped)

1 cup of watercress leaves

1 cucumber (diced)

2 tbsp fresh dill (finely chopped)

¼ red onion (chopped)

5-10 sliced olives

¼ red bell pepper (chopped)

¼ green bell pepper (chopped)

1 tbsp 100% date sugar syrup

3 tbsp water

⅛ tsp of sea salt

Directions:

1. Mix the date sugar syrup, water, and salt together

2. Mix all the remaining ingredients together in a bowl.

3. Massage in date syrup mix with the vegetables. Toss and serve.

NUT MILK

Almond, Brazil Nut, Hempseed, or Walnut Milk

Makes 5 cups
Ingredients:
1 cup of your selected nuts or seeds
4 cups water
2-3 pitted dates (optional)
sea salt (optional to taste)

Directions:
1. Add 1 cup water and nuts or seeds to blender. Using a high speed blender, blend for 2 minutes. Add in the remaining water and blend until liquefied. You may need to blend longer using a consumer blender.
2. You can strain the contents using a strainer and cheese cloth for a smooth milk, or you can leave all the contents for a hearty milk containing more nutrients.
3. Add milk back to blender with dates and blend for a sweeter milk.
4. Store in glass in fridge for up to 3 days.
5. If you decide to strain the milk you can add the discarded nuts or seeds to your vegetable juices.

CHEESE

Brazil Nut Cheese

Makes 3 cups
Ingredients:
8 oz. brazil nuts (soak overnight for creamier cheese)
¾ cup of hemp milk
¾ cup of water
¼ tsp of lime juice
1 tsp coconut oil
1 tsp sea salt
½ tsp onion powder
¼ tsp cayenne pepper
⅛ tsp rosemary

Directions:
1. Add all of the ingredients to the blender with only half the water. Blend for 1-2 minutes. You want the ingredients to turn in on each other instead of being spread apart with all the water
2. Add in the remaining water and blend to your desired consistency.

Makes a great vegetable dip.

TEAS

Drinking herbal tea is a great way to warm the body up, get more water into the body, and also a way to benefit from the healing nutrients of the herb. In many cases we discard the tea bag or strain the loose herb after the tea is made.

To get the full potency of the herb consider either consuming the ground herb with the tea, or mix the remaining herb with some water and drink it also.

Elderberry Tea

Used in traditional medicine to protect against flu and colds.

Makes 1 cup
Ingredients:
1 tbsp of dried elderberries
8 oz. of water
½ tbsp of date sugar (optional)

Directions:
1. Add water and elderberries to a saucepan, cover saucepan, bring to a boil, reduce heat to a simmer for 15 minutes.
2. This allows for the deep extraction of nutrients and phytonutrients from the elderberries into the water.
3. Remove from the heat, and strain into cup.
4. Add sugar if needed.
5. Let cool for 5 minutes.

Soursop Tea

Used in traditional medicine to protect against uric acid buildup (gout) and cancer.

Makes 1 cup
Ingredients:
1 soursop tea bag, or 3 soursop leaves cut into ¼ inch or smaller strips
8 oz. of water
¼ tsp of key lime juice
½ tbsp of date sugar (optional)

Directions:
1. Add water and soursop to a saucepan and bring to a boil, reduce heat to a simmer for 15 minutes.
2. This allows for the deep extraction of nutrients and phytonutrients from the soursop leaves into the water.
3. Remove from the heat, and strain into cup.
4. Add lime juice.
5. Add sugar if needed.
6. Let cool for 5 minutes.

Ginger Root Tea

Used in traditional medicine to protect against headaches, upset stomach, nausea and inflammation.

Makes 1 cup
Ingredients:
½ inch washed ginger root, sliced
8 oz. of water
½ tbsp of date sugar (optional)

Directions:

1. Add water and ginger root to a saucepan, cover pan, bring to a boil, reduce heat to a simmer for 15 minutes.

2. This allows for the deep extraction of nutrients and phytonutrients from the ginger root into the water.

3. Remove from the heat, and strain into cup.

4. Add date sugar if needed.

5. Let cool for 5 minutes.

Red Raspberry Leaf Tea

Used in traditional medicine to protect against diarrhea, flu, fever, and has been used by women to ease painful and heavy menstruation, and to strengthen the uterus.

Makes 1 cup

Ingredients:

1 teabag red raspberry, or 1 tbsp of crushed dried red raspberry leaves

8 oz. of water

½ tbsp of date sugar (optional)

Directions:

1. Add water to a saucepan, bring to a boil, and remove from heat.

2. Add raspberry and nettle leaves to water and let steep for 5 minutes.

3. Remove from the heat, and strain into cup.

4. Add date sugar if needed.

5. Let cool if needed.

Dandelion Root or Leaf Tea

Both the root and leaf are used in traditional medicine to protect and clean the liver and kidneys, though nutrients are more concentrated in the root, which is used more specifically to target the liver. Dandelion is a diuretic and strips the body of water by promoting urination. It is important to drink a recommended 1 gallon a day of water when taking diuretics.

Makes 1 cup
Ingredients:
1 tea bag dandelion leaf, or 1 tbsp of crushed dry leaves, or ¼ tsp of ground dandelion root
8 oz. of water
¼ tsp lime juice

Directions:
1. Add water to a saucepan, bring to a boil, and remove from heat.
2. Add bag, leaves, or ground root to water and let steep for 5 minutes.
3. Remove from the heat, and strain into cup, and let cool.

I Am Woman Tea

Makes 2 cups
Ingredients:
1 teabag red raspberry, or 1 tbsp of crushed dried red raspberry leaves
1 teabag nettle, or 1 tbsp of crushed dried nettle leaves
8 oz. of water
¼ tsp lime juice
½ tbsp of date sugar (optional)

Directions:
1. Add water to a saucepan, bring to a boil, and remove from heat.
2. Add bag, leaves, or root to water and let steep for 5 minutes.
3. Remove from the heat, and strain into cup, and let cool.

Me Man Tea

Used in traditional medicine to enhance libido.

Makes 2 cups
Ingredients:
¼ tsp of ground yohimbe bark
¼ tsp sarsaparilla root
16 oz. of water

Directions:
1. Add water, yohimbe bark and sarsaparilla to a saucepan, bring to a boil, then simmer for 15 minutes.
2. Remove from the heat, strain into cup, and let cool.

CHAPTER 18:

BACK TO GOD/THE SOURCE/NATURE

The reality is we are out of sync with the world, and this has very serious implications! There is a dependent relationship people have with the earth that is ignored to satisfy greed and gluttony. The pollution that industry causes depletes the ozone layer and diminishes the balance put in place by God/The Source/Nature to protect life on earth from excessive radiation exposure from the sun. This causes people to run from the sun that provides people with what might be the most important vitamin in supporting homeostasis, vitamin D.

Climate change is a very serious issue that is causing severe drought in the western United States, and studies predict a megadrought to occur over the next thirty-five years in the Southwest and Great Plains areas of the United States. It will last longer and be more severe than any other droughts that have occurred in the last thousand years. The research showed that natural patterns of drought are now being amplified and extended because of the excessive use of water and greenhouse gases being released into the environment. The number-one offender of water usage and the release of greenhouse gases into the environment is the meat industry.

Though industry is directly responsible for this negative impact on the natural patterns established by God/The Source/Nature, the responsibility ultimately lies with individual people. Yes, industry manipulates people into buying its products. Yes, a process that can see the big picture more clearly than most people manipulates people. In the end, individual people make things the way they are, because people buy the products and determine which industries we support.

Whether supporting products and industry that destroy the natural patterns that God/The Source/Nature is done intentionally or out of ignorance, it is still done. The collective actions of individuals are destroying the spiritual and supportive connections between the earth and people. Are we truly religious when we destroy our own bodies and support industries that destroy the earth's ecosystem that designed by God/The Source/Nature? Outside of religion, can we truly say we are spiritual beings when, through our individual actions, we destroy our own bodies and we support industries that destroy the earth's ecosystem designed by God/The Source/Nature? When we look at the spiritual and moral decline that is being globalized throughout the world, we need to look at how individual actions support the decline. People make dietary decisions that destroy the human body, the temple of God/The Source/Nature, which removes the spiritually and naturally patterned connection to life. This has the repercussion of building and supporting industries that destroy the earth's ecosystem and the life it supports.

ABOUT ME

My journey has been one of introspection and enlightenment. Enlightenment is attained through understanding and being in tune with the connectivity of all of life. This is truly a profound outlook on life because it takes focus off the ego and places focus on the beautiful patterns that sustain life. Total focus on the ego individualizes one's journey through life and fosters separation and illness.

I attained a BA in organizational behavior and communications from NYU. A major part of the curriculum involved understanding what culture was, how it developed and shaped people, and what unconscious norms people picked up and perpetuated, whether they were good or bad norms. The curriculum also involved learning how to address and change the norms that were detrimental to the individual and to the community. I also worked in social work and in education for a time, which helped me to really see and understand how patterns in society direct the development of individuals and communities for the good and for the bad.

A great personal change came into my life when I adopted a plant-based diet. Adopting a plant-based diet took discipline, but it also brought with it ease, patience, energy, clarity, youth, strength, endurance, health, and mental and emotional stability. It made me realize how much the body influences mental and emotional stability. Self-control is not only gained through willpower. It is equally influenced by the positive flow of energy that is linked to the health of the entire body. I am grateful for the enlightenment my plant-based diet has revealed to me, because it allowed me to strengthened my body, mind, and spirit. It also made me clearly see all life is interdependent and that is it very urgent that we wake up and realize this before the earth's ecosystem stops supporting life.

NOTES

1. Ed Yong, "Birds That Fly in a V Formation Use An Amazing Trick," *National Geographic*, June 31 2014, http://phenomena.nationalgeographic.com/2014/01/15/birds-that-fly-in-a-v-formation-use-an-amazing-trick/.

2. "Photosynthesis," The University of Illinois at Chicago, September 10, 2014. http://www.uic.edu/classes/bios/bios100/lecturesf04am/lect10.htm.

3. "Homeostasis In The Human Body," *Natural Life Energy*, February 20, 2015, http://www.naturallifeenergy.com/homeostasis-in-the-human-body/.

4. T. Colin Campbell Foundation and TILS, "Nutrition TCC501: Nutrition Fundamentals: On Nutrients And Their Interactions," Certificate Program in Plant-Based Nutrition (2012):1–2.

5. Mary Anne Dunkin, "Vitamin D Deficiency," *Web MD*, May 27, 2015, http://www.webmd.com/food-recipes/vitamin-d-deficiency.

6. "Ozone Depletion," *National Geographic*, March 23, 2015, http://environment.nationalgeographic.com/environment/global-warming/ozone-depletion-overview/.

7. "The Causes of Ozone Depletion," *BC Air Quality*, March 23, 2015, http://www.bcairquality.ca/101/ozone-depletion-causes.html.

8. "Health and Environmental Effects of Ozone Layer Depletion," *Environmental Protection Agency,* March 23, 2015, http://www.epa.gov/spdpublc/science/effects/index.html.

9. T. Osborn, "Amino Acids in Nutrition and Growth," *J Biol Chem* 17 (1914): 325.

10. T. Colin Campbell Foundation and TILS, "TCC501: Nutrition Fundamentals: On Protein Quality and Quantity," Certificate Program in Plant-Based Nutrition (2012):2.

11. T. Colin Campbell Foundation and TILS, "Nutrition TCC501: Nutrition Fundamentals: On Nutrients And Their Interactions."

12. "Position of the American Dietetic Association: Vegetarian Diets," *Vegetarian Nutrition*, September 1, 2015, http://vegetariannutrition.net/wp-content/uploads/2012/09/PositionPaperVegetarianDiets-909.pdf.

13. "Protein and Amino Acid Requirements in Human Nutrition," *World Health Organization Joint FAO/WHO/UNU Expert Consultation (2002)*: Table 50, p. 246, March 3, 2014. http://whqlibdoc.who.int/trs/WHO_TRS_935_eng.pdf.
14. T. Colin Campbell Foundation and TILS, "TCC502: Diet and Cancer II: Initiation versus Promotion." Certificate Program in Plant-Based Nutrition (2012):7.
15. T. Colin Campbell Foundation and TILS, "TCC501: Nutrition Fundamentals: On Protein Quality and Quantity."
16. T. Colin Campbell Foundation and TILS, "TCC501: Nutrition Fundamentals: Introduction to the Scientific Method." Certificate Program in Plant-Based Nutrition (2012):2–4.
17. T. Colin Campbell Foundation and TILS, "TCC501: Nutrition Fundamentals: Introduction to the Scientific Method."
18. T. Colin Campbell Foundation and TILS, "TCC501: Nutrition Fundamentals: Introduction to the Scientific Method."
19. Aqiyl Henry, "What are Phytonutrients and How do They Work in The Body?" *Natural Life Energy*, February 21, 2015, http://www.naturallifeenergy.com/what-are-phytonutrients-and-how-do-they-work-in-the-body/.
20. T. Colin Campbell Foundation and TILS, "TCC502: Diet and Cancer I: Chemical Causes of Cancer," Certificate Program in Plant-Based Nutrition (2012):3.
21. T. Colin Campbell Foundation and TILS, "TCC501: Nutrition Fundamentals: Introduction to the Scientific Method."
22. T. Colin Campbell Foundation and TILS, "TCC501: Nutrition Fundamentals: Introduction to the Scientific Method."
23. T. Colin Campbell Foundation and TILS, "TCC502: Diet and Cancer II: Initiation verses Promotion," Certificate Program in Plant-Based Nutrition (2012):10.
24. Mark Bittman, "Rethinking the Meat-Guzzler," *The New York Times*, December 15, 2014, http://www.nytimes.com/2008/01/27/weekinreview/27bittman.html.
25. "Factory Farming: Cruelty to Animals," *Peta*, September 21, 2014, http://www.peta.org/issues/animals-used-for-food/factory-farming/.
26. Paul McCartney, "Official 'Glass Walls' Video," *YouTube*, July 13, 2014, https://www.youtube.com/watch?v=ql8xkSYvwJs.
27. "Cows Fed Candy Instead of Corn On Kentucky Ranch Affected By Drought," *Huffington Post*, June 16, 2014, http://www.huffingtonpost.com/2012/08/21/cows-fed-candy-drought_n_1819366.html.
28. "Cash-strapped Farmers Feed Candy to Cows," *CNNMoney*, June 16, 2014, http://money.cnn.com/2012/10/10/news/economy/farmers-cows-candy-feed/.
29. "Mercury in Corn Syrup?" *Nutrition Facts.org*, July 1, 2014, http://nutritionfacts.org/video/mercury-in-corn-syrup/.
30. "Mercury in Corn Syrup?" *Nutrition Facts.org*. July 1, 2014, http://articles.mercola.com/sites/articles/archive/2009/04/21/msg-is-this-silent-

killer-lurking-in-your-kitchen-cabinets.aspx.

31. "High Cholesterol," *Mayo Clinic*. August 14, 2014,
http://www.mayoclinic.org/diseases-conditions/high-blood-cholesterol/in-depth/trans-fat/art-20046114.

32. "Nutrition and Healthy Eating." *Mayo Clinic*. August 14, 2014.
http://www.mayoclinic.org/healthy-living/nutrition-and-healthy-eating/expert-answers/phenylalanine/faq-20058361.

33. "Sawdust for Emergency Feeding of Dairy Cattle." *Penn State College of Agricultural Science*, February 12, 2014,
http://extension.psu.edu/prepare/emergencyready/drought/dairylivestock/sawdust.

34. "Southeast Iowa Cattle Herd Thriving on Sawdust-based Feed," *The Gazette*, February 12, 2014, http://thegazette.com/2013/02/25/northeast-iowa-cattle-herd-thriving-on-sawdust-based-feed/.

35. Michael Greger, "Mad Cow California: Stop Feeding Cows Chicken Manure," *Huffington Post*, March 2, 2014, http://www.huffingtonpost.com/michael-greger-md/mad-cow-disease-california_b_1450994.html.

36. "Feeding Poultry Litter to Beef Cattle," *Universtity of Missouri*, March 2, 2014, http://extension.missouri.edu/p/G2077.

37. "Diet, Escherichia coli O157:H7, and cattle: a review after 10 years." US National *Library of Medicine National Institutes of Health: Pub Med*, March 23, 2014, http://www.ncbi.nlm.nih.gov/pubmed/19351974.

38. Michael Pollan, *The Omnivore's Dilemma: A Natural History of Four Meals*, New York: Penguin, 2006,
http://books.google.com/books?id=Qh7dkdVsbDkC&printsec=frontcover&dq=the+omnivore%27s+dilemma&hl=en&sa=X&ei=NXR6Uu_nNMPIsASPzYLQBw&ved=0CEMQ6AEwAA - v=onepage&q=e. coli&f=false.

39. "5 Modern Diseases Grown by Factory Farming," *The Week*, March 23, 2014, http://theweek.com/articles/457135/5-modern-diseases-grown-by-factory-farming.

40. "MRSA and Animals FAQ," *American Veterinary Medical Association*, March 19, 2014, https://www.avma.org/KB/Resources/FAQs/Pages/MRSA-HHP-FAQs.aspx.

41. "The Hidden Health Hazards of Factory Farms," *Mother Earth News*, March 19, 2014, http://www.motherearthnews.com/natural-health/health-hazards-factory-farms-zmaz09fmzraw.aspx?PageId=5 - axzz2jnd1i4ID.

42. "Campylobacter," *Centers for Disease Control and Prevention*, February 19, 2014, http://www.cdc.gov/nczved/divisions/dfbmd/diseases/campylobacter/.

43. "Drug-resistant Campylobacter," *Centers for Disease Control and Prevention*. 19 February 2014, http://www.cdc.gov/drugresistance/threat-report-2013/pdf/ar-threats-2013-508.pdf - page=61.

44. "How Safe is That Chicken?" *Consumer Reports*, January 2010, http://www.consumerreports.org/cro/magazine-archive/2010/january/food/chicken-safety/overview/chicken-safety-ov.htm.
45. Michael Greger, "The Human/Animal Interface: Emergence and Resurgence of Zoonotic Infectious Diseases," *Critical Reviews in Microbiology* 33 (2007): 278, http://www.birdflubook.org/resources/Greger_2007_CRM_33(4)_243.pdf.
46. "Food Choices and the Planet," *Earth Save*. March 3, 2014, http://www.earthsave.org/environment.htm.
47. Mark Bittman, "Rethinking the Meat-Guzzler," *New York Times*, May 5, 2014, http://www.nytimes.com/2008/01/27/weekinreview/27bittman.html.
48. "Food Choices and the Planet," *Earth Save*. March 3, 2014. http://www.earthsave.org/environment.htm.
49. Robert Repetto, "Renewable Resources and Population Growth," *Population and Environment*, 10:4 (Summer 1989): 228–29, cited in Rifkin, Beyond Beef (New York: Dutton Press, 1992).
50. Myra Klockenbrink, "The New Range War Has the Desert as Foe," *New York Times*, August 20, 1991.
51. T. Colin Campbell Foundation and TILS, "TCC503: Environment I: The Environmental Impact of Food Production Part 1," Certificate Program in Plant-Based Nutrition (2012):11.
52. T. Colin Campbell Foundation and TILS, "TCC503: Environment II: The Environmental Impact of Food Production Part II," Certificate Program in Plant-Based Nutrition (2012):6–20.
53. T. Colin Campbell Foundation and TILS, "TCC503: Environment I: The Environmental Impact of Food Production Part 1," Certificate Program in Plant-Based Nutrition (2012):12.
54. "Unprecedented 21st Century Drought Risk in the American Southwest and Central Plains," *Science Advances*, March 5, 2014, http://advances.sciencemag.org/content/1/1/e1400082.
55. "Irrigation & Water Use," *United States Department of Agriculture*, March 5, 2014. http://www.ers.usda.gov/topics/farm-practices-management/irrigation-water-use.aspx.
56. David Pimentel and Marcia Pimentel, "Sustainability of meat-based and plant-based diets and the environment 1,2,3," *The American Journal of Clinical Nutrition* 78 (2003): 660S–3S.
57. T. Colin Campbell Foundation and TILS, "TCC503: Environment I: The Environmental Impact of Food Production Part I," Certificate Program in Plant-Based Nutrition (2012):7.
58. Mark Bittman, "Rethinking the Meat-Guzzler," *New York Times*, May 5, 2014, http://www.nytimes.com/2008/01/27/weekinreview/27bittman.html.
59. Mark Bittman, "Accessing the Environmental Impacts of Consumption and Production," *United Nations Environmental Programme*, May 15, 2014,

http://www.unep.org/resourcepanel/Portals/24102/PDFs/PriorityProductsAndM
aterials_Report.pdf.

60. T. Colin Campbell Foundation and TILS, "TCC503: Understanding and
Interpreting Scientific Research II: What Shapes the Evidence We Receive?"
Certificate Program in Plant-Based Nutrition (2012):9.

61. "ChooseMyPlate," *United States Department of Agriculture*, May 17, 2014,
http://www.choosemyplate.gov/.

62. "Court Rules Against USDA's Secrecy and Failure to Disclose Conflict of
Interest in Setting Nutrition Policies," Physicians Committee for Responsible
Medicine, October 2, 2000, http://www.pcrm.org/media/news/court-rules-
against-usdas-secrecy-and-failure-to.

63. "Dietary Reference Intakes for Energy, Carbohydrate, Fiber, Fat, Fatty Acids,
Cholesterol, Protein, and Amino Acids," *Institute of Medicine of the National
Academies* (2002), March 16, 2014, http://www.iom.edu/reports/2002/dietary-
reference-intakes-for-energy-carbohydrate-fiber-fat-fatty-acids-cholesterol-
protein-and-amino-acids.aspx.

64. T. Colin Campbell Foundation and TILS, "TCC501: Nutrition Fundamentals: On
Protein Quality and Quantity," Certificate Program in Plant-Based Nutrition
(2012):5.

65. "Protein," *Centers for Disease Control and Prevention*, March 16, 2014,
http://www.cdc.gov/nutrition/everyone/basics/protein.html.

66. "Diet, Nutrition, and Cancer Report," *The National Academies Press* (1982):4,
May 15, 2014, http://www.nap.edu/openbook.php?isbn=0309032806.

67. T. Colin Campbell Foundation and TILS, "TCC503: Understanding and
Interpreting Scientific Research III: Industry and Public Policy" Certificate Program
in Plant-Based Nutrition (2012):6.

68. Goran Bjelakovic, "Mortality in randomized trials of antioxidant supplements
for primary and secondary prevention: systematic review and meta-analysis,"
JAMA 297, no. 8 (2007): 842–57.

69. "Vitamins & Supplements," *WebMD*, December 20, 2014,
http://www.webmd.com/vitamins-and-supplements/news/20131216/experts-
dont-waste-your-money-on-multivitamins.

70. "Do supplements really work?," *ConsumerReports*, November 4, 2014,
http://www.consumerreports.org/cro/2014/05/do-vitamin-supplements-
work/index.htm.

71. T. Colin Campbell Foundation and TILS, "TCC501: Nutrition Fundamentals:
Design and Methodology of the China Project," Certificate Program in Plant-
Based Nutrition (2012).

72. "Homeostasis In The Human Body," *Natural Life Energy,* February 20, 2015,
http://www.naturallifeenergy.com/homeostasis-in-the-human-body/.

73. T. Colin Campbell Foundation and TILS, "Nutrition TCC501: Nutrition
Fundamentals: On Nutrients And Their Interactions," Certificate Program in Plant-

Based (2012):1–2.
74. "Blood Gases," *MedlinePlus*, March 21, 2015,
http://www.nlm.nih.gov/medlineplus/ency/article/003855.htm.
75. "Blood, Sweat, and Buffers: pH Regulation During Exercise," *Department of Chemistry, Washington University*, March 21, 2015,
http://www.chemistry.wustl.edu/~edudev/LabTutorials/Buffer/Buffer.html.
76. "Blood pH," *Harper College*, March 21, 2015,
http://www.harpercollege.edu/tm-ps/chm/100/dgodambe/thedisk/bloodbuf/zback.htm.
77. "Nutrition Facts," *NutritionFacts.org*. February 20, 2015,
http://nutritionfacts.org/.
78. Charles A. Janeway et al., *Immunobiology*, 5th edition: The Immune System in Health and Disease, New York: Garland Science; 2001,
http://www.ncbi.nlm.nih.gov/books/NBK27169/.
79. T. Colin Campbell Foundation and TILS, "TCC501: Nutrition Fundamentals: Introduction to the Scientific Method," Certificate Program in Plant-Based Nutrition (2012): 2–4.
80. J. Bartley and S. R. McGlashan, "Does Milk Increase Mucus Production?" *Medical Hypotheses* 74, no. 4 (2010): 732–4.
81. "Is Milk and Mucus a Myth?" *NutritionFacts.org*, March 17, 2014,
http://nutritionfacts.org/video/is-milk-and-mucus-a-myth/.
82. Dr. Victor Marcial-Vega, "Blood Before Goji After Goji" online video clip, *YouTube,* September 9, 2010,
https://www.youtube.com/watch?v=40mvty0EM2o.
83. Aqiyl Henry, "Goji Berries: What Are Goji Berries And Their Benefits?" *Natural Life Energy*, May19, 2013, http://www.naturallifeenergy.com/superfood-goji-berries-goji-berry-juice/.
84. "Calcium and Strong Bones" *Physicians Committee for Responsible Medicine*, March 21, 2014, http://www.pcrm.org/health/health-topics/calcium-and-strong-bones.
85. K. K. Frick et al., "Metabolic acidosis increases intracellular calcium in bone cells through activation of the proton receptor OGR1," *US National Library of Medicine National Institutes of Health*, November 13, 2013.
http://www.ncbi.nlm.nih.gov/pubmed/18847331.
86. Timothy R. Arnett, "Extracellular pH Regulates Bone Cell Function 1–3," *The Journal of Nutrition*, November 13, 2013.
http://jn.nutrition.org/content/138/2/415S.full.
87. "Multivitamins are, at Best, a Waste of Money, Johns Hopkins Doctors Say," *Johns Hopkins*, March 4, 2013, http://hub.jhu.edu/2013/12/17/vitamins-might-be-harmful.
88. "Don't Take Your Vitamins," *New York Times*, March 4, 2013.
http://www.nytimes.com/2013/06/09/opinion/sunday/dont-take-your-

vitamins.html?_r=0.

89. "The Nutrition Source," *Harvard T.H. Chan School of Public Health*, May 23, 2014, http://www.hsph.harvard.edu/nutritionsource/omega-3-fats/.

90. Stephanie Dutchen, "What Do Fats Do in the Body?" *Live Science*, May 23, 2014, http://www.livescience.com/9109-fats-body.html.

91. Stephanie Dutchen, "What Do Fats Do in the Body?" *Live Science*, May 23, 2014, http://www.livescience.com/9109-fats-body.html.

92. "Herbalist Found Not Guilty in Fake Healing Case," *Natural Life Energy,* February 25, 2014, http://www.naturallifeenergy.com/documents/sebi-found-not-guilty.pdf.

93. "CBS NEWS: The Man That Cures all Diseases," *Live Leak*, May 23, 2014, http://www.liveleak.com/view?i=9a1_1343602546.

94. "Your Brain On Pork! Pork Parasites Are Number One Cause Of Epilepsy," *Natural Life Energy,* December 15, 2014, http://www.naturallifeenergy.com/brain-pork-parasites-number-one-cause-epilepsy/.

95. Michael Greger, "Pork Tapeworms on the Brain," Online video clip, *YouTube,* September 9, 2013, https://www.youtube.com/watch?v=hhgXukqla5U.

96. "A Natural Approach to Migraines," *Physicians Committee for Responsible Medicine*, December 4, 2013, http://www.pcrm.org/health/health-topics/a-natural-approach-to-migraines.

97. Aqiyl Henry, "Alkaline Diet—Mucus Reducing Nutritional Guide," *Natural Life Energy,* May 17, 2013, http://www.naturallifeenergy.com/alkaline-producing-mucus-reducing-nutrional-guide/.

98. Peter Hedden et al., "Green Revolution Genes," *Plant Physiology Online*, November 14, 2013, http://5e.plantphys.net/article.php?id=355.

99. H. Ellis et al., ""Perfect" Markers for the Rht-B1b and Rht-D1b Dwarfing Genes in Wheat," *US National Library of Medicine National Institutes of Health*, November 14, 2013, http://www.ncbi.nlm.nih.gov/pubmed/12582931.

100. Aqiyl Henry, "What Is Processed Food? Is Processed Food Good Or Bad For You?" *Natural Life Energy,* May 23, 2013, http://www.naturallifeenergy.com/what-are-processed-foods-good-bad/.

101. "Trans Fat Now Listed With Saturated Fat and Cholesterol," *US Food and Drug Administration*, May 5, 2014, http://www.fda.gov/food/ingredientspackaginglabeling/labelingnutrition/ucm274590.htm.

102. "Effect of animal and industrial trans fatty acids on HDL and LDL cholesterol levels in humans—a quantitative review," *US National Library of Medicine National Institutes of Health*, June 17, 2014, http://www.ncbi.nlm.nih.gov/pubmed/20209147.

103. "Effect of Different Forms of Dietary Hydrogenated Fats on LDL Particle Size 1,2,3," *The American Journal of Clinical Nutrition*, June 17, 2014,

http://ajcn.nutrition.org/content/78/3/370.long.

104. Aqiyl Henry, "What is Cholesterol? Cholesterol Benefits," *Natural Life Energy,* June 17, 2014, http://www.naturallifeenergy.com/what-is-cholesterol-cholesterol-benefits/.

105. "Trans Fats," *American Heart Association*, June 17, 2014, http://www.heart.org/HEARTORG/GettingHealthy/NutritionCenter/HealthyEating/Trans-Fats_UCM_301120_Article.jsp.

106. "Trans Fatty Acids and Coronary Heart Disease," *Departments of Nutrition and Epidemiology, Harvard School of Public Health*, June 17, 2014, http://www.tfx.org.uk/docs/hsph_transfats.pdf.

107. "What is heart disease?" *Medical News Today*, June 17, 2014, http://www.medicalnewstoday.com/articles/237191.php.

108. "LDL Cholesterol: The Bad Cholesterol," *WebMD: Cholesterol & Triglycerides Health Center*, June 17, 2014, http://www.webmd.com/cholesterol-management/ldl-cholesterol-the-bad-cholesterol.

109. "Trans Fat," *CDC Centers for Disease Control and Prevention*, February 13, 2014, http://www.cdc.gov/nutrition/everyone/basics/fat/transfat.html.

110. "Generally Recognized as Safe (GRAS)," *FDA: US Food and Drug Administration*, March 11, 2014, http://www.fda.gov/Food/IngredientsPackagingLabeling/GRAS/.

111. "Food Manufacturers Get to Decide if Their Own Additives Are Safe," *Nutrition Fact.org*, February 9, 2014, http://nutritionfacts.org/2015/03/19/food-manufacturers-get-to-decide-if-their-own-additives-are-safe/.

112. Michael Greger, "Who Determines if Food Additives are Safe?" Online video clip. *YouTube.* February 9, 2014, http://nutritionfacts.org/video/who-determines-if-food-additives-are-safe/.

113. "EWG Releases Dirty Dozen Guide to Food Additives," *Mercola*. February 9, 2014, http://articles.mercola.com/sites/articles/archive/2014/11/26/12-worst-food-additives.aspx.

114. Aqiyl Henry, "Juicing Fruits and Vegetables Removes Polyphenols Stuck To Fiber—Make Smoothies Instead," *Natural Life Energy,* October 30, 2014, http://www.naturallifeenergy.com/juicing-fruits-vegetables-removes-polyphenols-stuck-fiber-make-smoothies/.

115. Michael Greger, "Juicing Removes More Than Just Fiber," Online video clip. *YouTube*. October 29, 2014, https://www.youtube.com/watch?t=193&v=U6tyu1Df1d4.

116. "Phytonutrients," *USDA National Agricultural Library*, November 17, 2014, https://fnic.nal.usda.gov/food-composition/phytonutrients.

117. Michael Greger, "Phytonutrients," *Nutrition Facts.org*, November 17, 2014. http://nutritionfacts.org/topics/phytonutrients/.

118. "Phytonutrient FAQs," *USDA United States Department of Agriculture Agricultural Research Service*, November 17, 2014,

http://www.ars.usda.gov/aboutus/docs.htm?docid=4142.

119. "Metabolic Danger of High-Fructose Corn Syrup," *Life Extension Magazine*, April 11, 2014, http://www.lef.org/magazine/2008/12/Metabolic-Dangers-of-High-Fructose-Corn-Syrup/Page-01.

120. "Study Finds High-Fructose Corn Syrup Contains Mercury," *Washington Post*, April 11, 2014, http://www.washingtonpost.com/wp-dyn/content/article/2009/01/26/AR2009012601831.html.

121. "Watch Out: Corporations Have Renamed 'High-Fructose Corn Syrup,'" *Natural Society*, December 10, 2014, http://naturalsociety.com/watch-corporations-renamed-high-fructose-corn-syrup/.

122. Courtney Winston, "List of Refined Carbs," *SFGate*, December 10, 2014, http://healthyeating.sfgate.com/list-refined-carbs-7260.html.

123. "Glycogen Metabolism Notes," *Oregon State University*, December 8, 2014, http://oregonstate.edu/instruct/bb450/summer09/lecture/glycogennotes.html.

124. "Converting Carbohydrates to Triglycerides," *National Council of Strength and Fitness*, December 8, 2014. http://www.ncsf.org/enew/articles/articles-convertingcarbs.aspx.

125. "Resistant Starch: Promise for Improving Human Health 1,2," *Advance in Nutrition*, June 4, 2014, http://advances.nutrition.org/content/4/6/587.long.

126. Michael Greger, "Juicing Removes More Than Just Fiber," Online video clip. *YouTube*. October 29, 2014, https://www.youtube.com/watch?t=193&v=U6tyu1Df1d4.

127. "Resistant Starch: What is it? And Why is it so Good for You?" *Precision Nutrition*, April 14, 2014, http://www.precisionnutrition.com/all-about-resistant-starch.

128. Goran Bjelakovic, "Mortality in randomized trials of antioxidant supplements for primary and secondary prevention: systematic review and meta-analysis," *JAMA*. (2007): 297(8):842–57.

129. "Vitamins & Supplements," *WebMD*, December 20, 2014, http://www.webmd.com/vitamins-and-supplements/news/20131216/experts-dont-waste-your-money-on-multivitamins.

130. "Do supplements really work?" *ConsumerReports*, November 4, 2014, http://www.consumerreports.org/cro/2014/05/do-vitamin-supplements-work/index.htm.

131. "Guidance for Industry: Guide to Minimize Microbial Food Safety Hazards for Fresh Fruits and Vegetables," *US Department of Health and Human Services: Food and Drug Administration: Center for Food Safety and Applied Nutrition* (CFSAN), 1998. 10–19. April 23, 2014, http://www.fda.gov/downloads/Food/GuidanceRegulation/UCM169112.pdf.

132. "Vitamin B12 Fact Sheet for Consumers," *National Institutes of Health*, December 16, 2013, http://ods.od.nih.gov/factsheets/VitaminB12-Consumer/.

133. "The Vitamin B12 Issue," *Vibrancy*, December 16, 2013,

http://www.vibrancyuk.com/B12.html.

134. "Enterohepatic Circulation: Physiological, Pharmacokinetic and Clinical Implications," *US National Library of Medicine National Institutes of Health*, December 16, 2013, http://www.ncbi.nlm.nih.gov/pubmed/12162761.

135. "Vitamin B12 Deficiency," *WebMD*, March 3, 2014, http://www.webmd.com/food-recipes/guide/vitamin-b12-deficiency-symptoms-causes.

136. "Anemia—B12 Deficiency," *MedlinePlus*, March 3, 2014, http://www.nlm.nih.gov/medlineplus/ency/article/000574.htm.

137. "Are Intestinal Bacteria a Reliable Source of B12?" *Vegan Health.org*, March 3, 2014. http://www.nlm.nih.gov/medlineplus/ency/article/000574.htm.

138. T. Colin Campbell Foundation and TILS, "TCC503: The Role of Supplements," Certificate Program in Plant-Based Nutrition (2012):6.

139. P. Lips, "Vitamin D Physiology," *Prog Biophys Mol Biol* 92, no. 1 (2006): 4–8.

140. M. F. Holick, "Sunlight and Vitamin D for Bone Health and Prevention of Autoimmune Diseases, Cancers, and Cardiovascular Disease," *Am J Clin Nutr* 80, 6 Suppl. (2004):1678S–88S.

141. C. J. Rosen et al., "The Nonskeletal Effects of Vitamin D: an Endocrine Society Scientific Statement," *Endocr Rev* 33, no. 3 (2012):456–92. doi: 10.1210/er.2012-1000. May 17, 2012.

142. T. Colin Campbell Foundation and TILS, "TCC503: The Role of Supplements," Certificate Program in Plant-Based Nutrition (2012):7.

143. "Testing For Vitamin D," *Vitamin D Council*, May 5, 2014, https://www.vitamindcouncil.org/about-vitamin-d/testing-for-vitamin-d/.

144. "Evaluation, Treatment, and Prevention of Vitamin D Deficiency: An Endocrine Society Clinical Practice Guideline," *The Endocrine Society's Clinical Guidelines*, May 5, 2014, https://www.endocrine.org/~/media/endosociety/Files/Publications/Clinical Practice Guidelines/FINAL-Standalone-Vitamin-D-Guideline.pdf.

145. "Vitamin D," *National Institutes of Health*, May 5, 2014, http://ods.od.nih.gov/factsheets/VitaminD-HealthProfessional/.

146. "UV Index Scale," *EPA: United States Environmental Protection Agency*, August 13, 2014, http://www2.epa.gov/sunwise/uv-index-scale.

147. "Dermato Endocrinology: Solar UV Doses of Adult Americans and Vitamin D3 Production," *US National Library of Medicine National Institutes of Health*, March 13, 2014, http://www.ncbi.nlm.nih.gov/pmc/articles/PMC3256341/.

148. "What are Proteins and What Do They Do?" *Genetics Home Reference: A Service of the US National Library of Medicine*, May 23, 2014. http://ghr.nlm.nih.gov/handbook/howgeneswork/protein.

149. "Long Term Toxicity of a Roundup Herbicide and a Roundup-Tolerant Genetically Modified Maize," *Food and Chemical Toxicity*, May 4, 2014, http://www.naturallifeenergy.com/files/seralini-study.pdf.

150. "Scientists Fight Against Retraction of Séralini GMO Rat Study," *Natural Life Energy,* January 1, 2014, http://www.naturallifeenergy.com/scientists-fight-retraction-sralini-gmo-rat-study/.

151. T. Bohn et al., "Compositional Differences in Soybeans on the Market: Glyphosate Accumulates in Roundup Ready GM Soybeans," *Food Chem* 153 (2014): 207–15.

152. Michael Greger, "Are GMOs Safe? The Case of Roundup Ready Soy," *Nutrition Fact.org*, November 30, 2014, http://nutritionfacts.org/video/are-gmos-safe-the-case-of-roundup-ready-soy/.

153. N. Benachour et al., "Time-and Dose-Dependent Effects of Roundup on human Embryonic and Placental Cells," *Arch Environ Contam Toxicol* 53, no. 1 (2007): 126–33.

154. S. Richard et al., "Differential Effects of Glyphosate and Roundup on Human Placental Cells and Aromatase," *Environmental Health Perspectives* 113, no. 6 (2005): 716–20.

155. R. Mesnage et al., "Major Pesticides Are More Toxic to Human Cells Than Their Declared Active Principles," *Environmental Health Perspectives*, Biomed Research International, 2014: 179691.

156. T. Bohn et al., "Compositional Differences in Soybeans on the Market: Glyphosate Accumulates in Roundup Ready GM Soybeans," *Food Chem* 153 (2014): 207–15.

157. T. Colin Campbell Foundation and TILS, "TCC501: Nutrition Fundamentals: Design and Methodology of the China Project," Certificate Program in Plant-Based Nutrition (2012): 3.

158. "Omega-6 Fatty Acids," *University of Maryland Medical Center*, June 13, 2014, http://umm.edu/health/medical/altmed/supplement/omega6-fatty-acids.

159. Bruce McDonald, "Canola Oil Nutritional Properties," *Oklahoma State University: Department of Plant and Soil Properties*, June 13, 2014, http://canola.okstate.edu/canola-info/nutrition/Nutritionalprop.pdf.

160. T. Colin Campbell Foundation and TILS, "TCC501: Nutrition Fundamentals: Understanding Fats and Carbohydrates," Certificate Program in Plant-Based Nutrition (2012):2.

161. "Detoxify The Blood with Burdock Root," *Natural Life Energy,* August 5, 2014, http://www.naturallifeenergy.com/herbs-burdock-root/.

162. "Study Shows Black Seed Cured HIV Patient," *Natural Life Energy,* August 5, 2014, http://www.naturallifeenergy.com/study-showed-black-seed-cured-hiv-patient/.

163. "Bromelain and Papain Plant Enzymes Aid In The Digestion Of Proteins," *Natural Life Energy,* August 5, 2014, http://www.naturallifeenergy.com/bromelain-papain-plant-enzymes-digest-proteins/.

164. "Benefits of Papain—A Protein Digesting Enzyme," *Natural Life Energy,*

August 5, 2014, http://www.naturallifeenergy.com/benefits-of-papain-a-protein-digesting-enzyme/.
165. "What Is Chlorella and Why Do I Need It?" *Natural Life Energy,* August 5, 2014, http://www.naturallifeenergy.com/what-is-chlorella-good-for/.
166. "Turmeric Benefits | Curcumin Benefits | Anti-Inflammatory Joint and Brain Food," *Natural Life Energy,* August 5, 2014,
http://www.naturallifeenergy.com/turmeric-benefits-curcumin-benefits/.
167. "Dandelion Root Benefits and Dandelion Leaf Benefits," *Natural Life Energy,* August 5, 2014, http://www.naturallifeenergy.com/dandelion-herb-root-and-leaves-dandelion-benefits/.
168. "Elderberry Extract Is a Natural Way of Fighting Colds and Flu," *Natural Life Energy,* August 5, 2014, http://www.naturallifeenergy.com/elderberry-extract-is-a-natural-way-of-fighting-colds/.
169. "Mullein Leaf Clears Mucus from The Body," *Natural Life Energy,* August 5, 2014, http://www.naturallifeenergy.com/benefits-of-mullein-leaf-herb-in-clearing-mucus-from-the-body/.
170. "Sarsaparilla Benefits—Detoxify The Blood," *Natural Life Energy,* August 5, 2014, http://www.naturallifeenergy.com/benefits-of-mullein-leaf-herb-in-clearing-mucus-from-the-body/.
171. "Evaluation of the medicinal use of clay minerals as antibacterial agents," *US National Library of Medicine National Institutes of Health*, December 17, 2013, http://www.ncbi.nlm.nih.gov/pmc/articles/PMC2904249/.
172. "6 Health Benefits of Bentonite Clay," *Global Healing Center*, August 30, 2014, http://www.globalhealingcenter.com/natural-health/6-health-benefits-bentonite-clay/.
173. "Diverticulosis and Diverticulitis," Medline Plus. August 30, 2014, http://www.nlm.nih.gov/medlineplus/diverticulosisanddiverticulitis.html.
174. "Psyllium," *University of Maryland Medical Center*, August 4, 2014, http://umm.edu/health/medical/altmed/supplement/psyllium.
175. "Dietary Reference Intakes: Water, Potassium, Sodium, Chloride, and Sulfate," *Institute of Medicine*, September 3, 2014,
https://www.iom.edu/Reports/2004/Dietary-Reference-Intakes-Water-Potassium-Sodium-Chloride-and-Sulfate.aspx.
176. A. Ermund et al., "Studies of Mucus in Mouse Stomach, Small Intestine, and Colon. I. Gastrointestinal Mucus Layers Have Different Properties Depending on Location as Well as Over the Peyer's Patches," *US National Library of Medicine National Institutes of Health*, March 15, 2014, http://www.ncbi.nlm.nih.gov/pubmed/23832518.
177. "Cleansing The Small Intestine," *WHALE*, September 14, 2014, http://www.whale.to/a/intestine.html.
178. "Kupffer Cell Heterogeneity: Functional Properties of Bone Marrow–Derived and Sessile Hepatic Macrophages," *US National Library of Medicine National*

Institutes of Health, January 5, 2014,
http://www.ncbi.nlm.nih.gov/pmc/articles/PMC2190614/.
179. "Alcoholic Liver Disease," *Medline Plus*, January 5, 2014,
http://www.nlm.nih.gov/medlineplus/ency/article/000281.htm.
180. "Diseases and Conditions: Liver Disease," *Mayo Clinic*, January 5, 2014,
http://www.mayoclinic.org/diseases-conditions/liver-problems/basics/risk-factors/con-20025300.
181. "Burdock," *University of Maryland Medical Center*, January 7, 2014,
http://umm.edu/health/medical/altmed/herb/burdock.
182. "Burdock," *Memorial Sloan Kettering Cancer Center*, January 7, 2014,
http://www.mskcc.org/cancer-care/herb/burdock.
183. Chung My Park et al., "Amelioration of Oxidative Stress by Dandelion Extract Through CYP2E1 Suppression Against Acute Liver Injury Induced by Carbon Tetrachloride in Sprague-Dawley Rats," *Phytotherapy Research* 24, no. 9 (2010): 1347–1353, http://onlinelibrary.wiley.com/doi/10.1002/ptr.3121/abstract.
184. "Yellow Dock," *WebMD*, March 17, 2014,
http://www.webmd.com/vitamins-supplements/ingredientmono-651-yellow dock.aspx?activeingredientid=651&activeingredientname=yellow dock.
185. "Sarsaparilla Benefits—Detoxify The Blood," Natural Life Energy, January 8, 2012, http://www.naturallifeenergy.com/herbs-sarsaparilla-benefits/.
186. "How to Clean Your Liver—Gallbladder | Liver—Gallbladder Cleanse," *Natural Life Energy*, December 5, 2014, http://www.naturallifeenergy.com/liver-gallbladder-cleanse/.
187. Michael Greger, "Kale and the Immune System," *Nutrition Facts.org*, November 2, 2013, http://nutritionfacts.org/video/kale-and-the-immune-system/.
188. "Kale, Raw," *Self Nutrition Data*, November 2, 2013,
http://nutritiondata.self.com/facts/vegetables-and-vegetable-products/2461/2.
189. "Mercury Detoxification Protocol," *Dr. Mercola.com*. December 14, 2013, https://www.mercola.com/article/mercury/detox_protocol.htm.
190. "Cilantro and Chlorella Can Remove 80% of Heavy Metals from the Body within 42 Days," *Natural Society*, December 14, 2013,
http://naturalsociety.com/proper-heavy-metal-chelation-cilantro-chlorella/.
191. "The Amazing and Mighty Ginger," *Herbal Medicine: Biomolecular and Clinical Aspects*, 2nd Edition, March 4, 2014,
http://www.ncbi.nlm.nih.gov/books/NBK92775/
192. "Ginger," *University of Maryland Medical Center*, December 14, 2013,
http://umm.edu/health/medical/altmed/herb/ginger.
193. M. Bortolotti et al., "The Treatment of Functional Dyspepsia with Red Pepper," *Aliment. Pharmacol. Ther* 16, no. 6 (2002): 1075–1082.
194. Michael Greger, "Cayenne Pepper for Irritable Bowel Syndrome and Chronic Indigestion," *Nutrition Facts.org*, February 9, 2014,

http://nutritionfacts.org/video/cayenne-pepper-for-irritable-bowel-syndrome-and-chronic-indigestion/.
195. "Investigation of the Effect of Ginger on the Lipid Levels. A Double Blind Controlled Clinical Trial," *US National Library of Medicine National Institutes of Health*, February 9, 2014, http://www.ncbi.nlm.nih.gov/pubmed/18813412.
196. "Omega-3 fatty acids," *University of Maryland Medical Center*, February 9, 2014, http://umm.edu/health/medical/altmed/supplement/omega3-fatty-acids.
197. "The Role of Vitamin C in Iron Absorption," *US National Library of Medicine National Institutes of Health*, March 4, 2014.
http://www.ncbi.nlm.nih.gov/pubmed/2507689.
198. "Effect of Ascorbic Acid Intake on Nonheme-Iron Absorption From a Complete Diet 1,2," *The American Journal of Clinical Nutrition*, March 4, 2014, http://ajcn.nutrition.org/content/73/1/93.full.
199. "The Water In You," *The USGS Water Science School*, May 3, 2014, https://water.usgs.gov/edu/propertyyou.html.
200. "Dehydration in Adults," *WebMD*, May 3, 2014, http://www.webmd.com/a-to-z-guides/dehydration-adults.

CPSIA information can be obtained
at www.ICGtesting.com
Printed in the USA
LVOW10s2054131017
552314LV00002B/18/P